DARE to be You

A Systems Approach to the Early Prevention
of Problem Behaviors

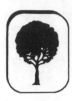

PREVENTION IN PRACTICE LIBRARY

SERIES EDITOR
Thomas P. Gullotta
Child and Family Agency, New London, Connecticut

ADVISORY BOARD
George W. Albee, University of Vermont
Evvie Becker, U.S. Department of Health and Human Services
Martin Bloom, University of Connecticut
Emory Cowen, University of Rochester
Roger Weissberg, University of Illinois
Joseph Zins, University of Cincinnati

DARE to be You

A Systems Approach to the Early Prevention
of Problem Behaviors

Jan Miller-Heyl
David MacPhee

and

Janet J. Fritz
Colorado State University
Fort Collins, Colorado

Kluwer Academic/Plenum Publishers
New York, Boston, Dordrecht, London, Moscow

Library of Congress Cataloging-in-Publication Data

Miller-Heyl, Janet L., 1944–
    DARE To Be You: A systems approach to the early prevention of problem behaviors/
Janet L. Miller-Heyl, David MacPhee, and Janet J. Fritz.
        p.   cm. — (Prevention in practice library)
    Includes bibliographical references and index.
    ISBN 0-306-46392-X (hardcover)—ISBN 0-306-46393-8 (pbk.)
        1. DARE to be You (Program)   2. Behavior disorders in children.   3. Behavior
disorders in children—Prevention.   4. Preschool children—Mental health.   I. MacPhee,
David, 1954–.   II. Fritz, Janet J., 1942–.   III. Title.   IV. Series.

RJ506.B44 M535 2001
618.92′8905—dc21

                                                                                    00-035239

ISBN 0-306-46392-X (Hardbound)
ISBN 0-306-46393-8 (Paperback)

©2001 Kluwer Academic / Plenum Publishers, New York
233 Spring Street, New York, New York 10013

http://www.wkap.nl/

10 9 8 7 6 5 4 3 2 1

A C.I.P. record for this book is available from the Library of Congress

Printed in the United States of America

DARE to be You

A Systems Approach to the Early Prevention of Problem Behaviors

Jan Miller-Heyl

David MacPhee

Janet J. Fritz

Preface

The growing concern about the bleak future of many youth has produced an explosion of programs designed to reduce problem behaviors and build assets (National Research Council, 1993). Concerned citizens who want to initiate community-based programs for youth must decide how to expend their resources in the most effective way. Some programs have a strong scientific basis and have also been proven to work (see Drug Strategies, 1999). Some have not. DARE to be You is a program that has both a conceptual foundation and is demonstrably effective in building assets that are linked to fewer problem behaviors. Its success is based on working not only with the individual child but also with multiple systems that affect the child. These systems include family, peers, school, and the broader community. Different contexts exert greater influence at some ages than others, so DARE to be You has devised age-appropriate curricula and adapted its overall approach to account for changing developmental needs.

The DARE to be You (DTBY) program builds the competencies of both the youth and the people who work with them. For youth, it provides both strategies and activities to enhance positive development and resilience. DTBY also provides a framework for developing positive environments for effective youth development.

The curriculum has components for individuals, families, schools, peers, and communities. Each of the components is based on ecological models of human development (e.g., Bronfenbrenner & Morris, 1998), social-cognitive theory (Bandura, 1986), and theories of reasoning about moral and social problems (e.g., Dodge, 1986; Piaget, 1965). The DTBY logo provides a simple way to remember key constructs of the program:

Decision-making, reasoning skills, and problem solving
Assertive communication and social skills
Responsibility (internal locus of control/attributions) and role models
Esteem, efficacy, and empathy

This monograph focuses on the DTBY program for families with 2- to 5-year-old youth. It also refers to the programs for school-aged children and teens.

The entire family is involved in the early prevention program for preschool-aged youth. Incentives encourage the involvement of several adult family members. Siblings are invited to special activities designed for their age group. The program also involves the schools and community by providing training for preschool and day care providers and agency staff that interact with the families. A primary focus of each component is the development of the competencies and efficacy of the adults and teens who work with the preschool-age youth. Parent efficacy, personal efficacy, and teaching efficacy are fostered. The program is designed to work with families for two or more years.

In the original 5-year demonstration project, four diverse sites in Colorado implemented the program to test its applicability across cultural and community settings. These sites included a Native American community in southwest Colorado; Colorado Springs, an urban setting of mixed cultures; the San Luis Valley, which is a traditional Hispanic and Anglo rural community; and Montezuma County, a poor, isolated agricultural region with Anglo, Native American, and Hispanic families.

Although families entered the program with varying degrees of risk and from different cultural systems, positive and statistically significant changes were similar at all sites. This indicates that the basic intervention processes can be adapted to diverse cultures and family backgrounds without sacrificing the integrity of DTBY. The original preschool/family program has also been replicated with positive outcomes in another Native American Tribe, six Asian Pacific Islander groups, and additional Hispanic populations.

THE IMPORTANCE OF PERSPECTIVE

One of my favorite paintings hangs in the National Museum of Art, Washington, DC. It is in the corner of a popular gallery but often receives only a glance from passersby. The temptation is to stand close to observe the carefully wrought spots of color. Each dot of color has been well thought out and carefully placed. Each section could stand alone. The patterns, meticulously wrought as they are, precise as they are, interesting as they are, could easily blind the viewer to the bigger picture. One must step back.

Then, the spots of paint reveal themselves as subtle variations of light and shade; they cohere into a gestalt of air, water, landscape, and a luminous lighthouse. The patterns of colored points suddenly make sense.

Seurat's pointillist lighthouse[1] is a warning beacon and a challenge to those who methodically examine narrowly drawn aspects of youth at risk. Though each

[1]The Lighthouse at Honfleur, Georges Seurat, 1886.

point is important, it is only part of the whole picture. If we are so absorbed with a certain piece of the pattern before us that we neglect to stand back, we miss the whole picture.

In this era when worrisome numbers of people, young and not young, are crashing on invisible reefs, we know that none of us alone has the entire picture. Our challenge is to join together to complete the picture as a beacon for those who follow.

If we dare to believe that our society can find the means to reduce the number of problem behaviors, we must adopt a broad, long-term vision of the complex factors that contribute to substance abuse, violence, poor educational outcomes, and other potentially harmful behaviors. Why are we concerned? The loss to individuals and families when people do not reach their potential is tragic. When these individual tragedies are multiplied, the cost to society is unbearable. More important, the legacy of damage we leave for future generations is inexcusable.

Prevention, as practiced in the 1980s and 1990s, expanded from a focus on strategies that directly affect substance abuse to include strategies that modify predictors of problem behaviors (Hansen, 1997; Reynolds, Stewart, & Fisher, 1997). Such approaches include reducing risk factors and building resiliency or, more recently, assets (Benson, Leffert, Scales, & Blyth, 1998). These factors are usually addressed through work with the individual, families, peer groups, and/or other related groups such as school, work, and communities. There has also been a change from a paternalistic pattern of seeing individuals as problems to be fixed to seeing people embedded in ecological systems and possessing many strengths (MacPhee, 1999).

Yet there is room for improvement in how prevention is put into practice:

- Important cross-system relationships may be ignored. Individuals, families, and schools may still be seen as separate from the broader community and society. The most effective prevention programs are ecological in design and effect (MacPhee, 1999; Schorr, 1989; Yoshikawa, 1994).
- Prevention programs that target a single process, such as peer refusal skills or reflective listening, are doomed to fail. Even if we focus on an entire family system and ignore broader contextual influences, we can fail. Risk factors have more than a cumulative effect; they interact with or potentiate each other (Rutter, 1979; Sameroff & Seifer, 1983). This means that model prevention programs must involve protection against multiple risks (Yoshikawa, 1994).
- Assets and risk factors are often considered in reference to the dominant culture. Therefore, assets based on traditional value systems may be overlooked. A "stable home life" is considered an asset. However, many Native American children are effectively raised by moving between grandparents', parents', and aunts' homes. Literature on the impact of different discipline strategies shows that authoritarian parenting may put children in

Anglo cultures at risk, but a similar pattern is not always seen in African-American populations (Deater-Deckard, Dodge, Bates, & Pettit, 1996).

- Often, problem behaviors such as alcohol and drug use are viewed as a youth problem. This bias can blind preventionists to the fact that addictions can start later in life or be maintained over the entire life span (Daughterty & Leukefeld, 1998). For instance, different risk factors may predispose people to early- versus late-onset substance abuse (Dobkin, Tremblay, & Sacchitelle, 1997) as well as antisocial behavior (Loeber, Green, Keenan, & Lahey, 1995; Moffitt, 1993). Also, substance abuse and conduct disorders tend to co-occur (Dobkin et al., 1997; Watson, Hancock, Gearhart, Malhovrh, Mendez, & Raden, 1997). They are both correlated with several of the same personality characteristics such as novelty or sensation seeking (Howard, Kivlahan, & Walker, 1997; Rowe & Rodgers, 1989), and both seem to be promoted when parents are more authoritarian and less consistent in their discipline (Dobkin et al., 1997). These results suggest that different screening procedures and intervention strategies are needed, depending on the disorder's age of onset.
- Prevention workers are often hesitant to consider spiritual influences as a resiliency factor (MacQueen, 1999). Strategies that increase hope, social cohesion, and social control—including those with a spiritual basis—can prove fruitful in preventing youths' substance use (McBride, Mutch, & Chitwood, 1996), especially when combined with parent monitoring of affiliation with deviant peers (Brownfield & Sorenson, 1991).
- Interventions are often structured with only the present situation in mind. This ignores the importance of developmental history, the salience of risk factors in different stages of life, and whether risk factors are chronic or acute. For example, long-term exposure to a hostile home environment is likely to require more intensive intervention, and program effects may take longer to emerge (Coie, Watt, West, Hawkins, Asarnow, Markman, Ramey, Shure & Long, 1993; Yoshikawa, 1994).

Despite these potential weaknesses in some prevention models, many have strengths that must be valued and used. One powerful approach is to work with multiple systems, which is discussed in the next chapter. This ecological approach, which draws from several theoretical traditions, provides more inclusive and meaningful mechanisms to address problem behaviors.

AS THE TWIG IS BENT

An old adage says, "A tree falls in the direction that it leans." It follows that saplings should be encouraged to adopt an upright posture from an early age. A core presumption of DTBY is that *early* intervention with at-risk families will have more impact and lasting benefits than waiting until youth begin to manifest problems with substance use, peer problems, and antisocial behavior. Several leading experts lighting the way have argued eloquently for greater attention to developing capable youth. For instance, Emmy Werner (1990) said that early intervention services "... need to focus especially on infants and young children who appear most vulnerable because they lack, temporarily or permanently, some of the essential social bonds that appear to buffer stress" (p. 112). More philosophically, James Garbarino (1992) asked, "Why care for children in the first place? Because they are the future. The continuing good of this earth and whatever is good on it depends on them" (pp. 305–306).

Research supports an emphasis on early prevention programs. From infancy, family processes may put children at risk for later substance use through poor management practices and permissive attitudes toward risk taking (see Hawkins, Catalano, & Miller, 1992). The same conclusion applies to antisocial behavior. Loeber and Dishion (1983) found that the earliest predictor of delinquency, and one of the strongest, was a composite of parenting styles and family functioning measured at age 6. In Patterson's model (Patterson, DeBaryshe, & Ramsey, 1989), conduct problems in middle childhood set the stage for peer rejection, school failure, substance use, and delinquency, but these conduct problems are shaped by parents who are poor disciplinarians from early childhood on. A panel convened for the National Prevention Conference (Coie et al., 1993) reviewed the evidence for early risk factors (see also National Research Council, 1993) and prevention programs. They concluded that a guiding principle in prevention science should be to address risk factors before they stabilize as predictors of dysfunction.

Early family-based prevention can promote developmental assets before critical risk factors can coalesce. This assertion rests on the following observations. First, behavioral genetics research suggests that a common, latent trait underlies a variety of deviant adolescent behaviors, from substance abuse and delinquency to school failure and precocious sexual intercourse (Rowe & Rodgers, 1989). Other reviews also document the co-occurrence of these deviant or risk-taking behaviors (e.g., Hawkins et al., 1992; Scales, 1990). Second, certain early protective and risk factors are common to many disorders that emerge in early adolescence. Among these protective factors are social skills, problem solving and critical thinking, a sense of purpose, social support, and family communication and conflict management (Coie et al., 1993; Scales, 1990; Werner, 1990), all of which reduce the risk of behavioral problems in adolescence. A common element in many of these resiliency factors is effective child rearing, which has led observers to call for greater investment in early childhood and parent support programs (Hawkins et al., 1992; Scales, 1990), as well as community-based initiatives that promote youth services and combat poverty.

In the next chapter, we elaborate on the argument that family-based programs need to be provided in tandem with interventions that focus on ecological systems such as social networks, schools, and community contexts. Our approach is consistent with the emerging view that comprehensive multisystem interventions, compared to those that are more limited in scope, are likely to have more impact on families. This is especially true if they enhance resilience while addressing risk factors (Cowan, Powell, & Cowan, 1998; Schorr, 1989). Such programs are particularly needed for multiple-risk families from diverse populations, but few of the widely disseminated parenting programs are empirically validated. Thus, we believe the DTBY program fills an important need for these families.

Acknowledgments

The DARE to be You program works because of the collective experience and knowledge of staff, community volunteers and supportive families. Special recognition needs to go to people who have been involved for at least three years and who have made substantial contributions: at the Ute Mountain Ute Head Start, Glenda Lopez; at the Colorado Springs Child Nursery Centers, Diane Price, Kim Fitzgerald, and Sally Ziegler; at the El Paso County Department of Health and Environment, Julie Davis; in the San Luis Valley Cooperative Extension, Jacque Miller and Tamara Grant; in the Montezuma County Site, Mari Martin, Jennie Preston, Gloria Balfour and in our central office, Sue Sidinger. Replication sites have added to our knowledge and we would like to recognize those that have contributed for at least three years. Special thanks go to those involved in the Navajo Replication site: Rose Woody, Ruby Hall and Deborah Nells. We appreciate Pam Thurston in the Pueblo site. The Head Start replication added knowledge about the impact on children: Thank you to Tracy Mandel, Judy Hite, Renee Podonovich, Eric Howey, and Mike Bonner.

Special appreciation for loving support and putting up with being "subjects," for testing many theories, for hours of volunteer help goes to: Keena and Aneka Miller, Bob Heyl, Darcy and Maura MacPhee, and the families of the staff.

Implementation of the DARE to be You curriculum as well as evaluation of its impact were supported in part by grants from the U.S. Department of Education (G00872063-87) and from the Center for Substance Abuse Prevention (High-Risk Youth Grant #1397). A special thanks is given to CSAP project officers, Tommie Johnson Waters and Stephen Gardner. Contracts and grants for program development were funneled through the Colorado State University Cooperative Extension Youth Development and the Department of Human Development and Family Studies. We express our gratitude to these entities for their sponsorship.

Contents

DARE to be You

A Systems Approach to the Early Prevention
of Problem Behaviors

Ecological Systems and Social–Cognitive Theory as a Basis for Building Resiliency

> When a person is part of a system, he cannot easily see what his role accomplishes ... Unless he understands the system thoroughly, he will not have any inkling of the network of controls that may or may not exist to keep the flow(s) continuous, adapted to inputs, adapted to outside demands, and stabilized in the face of fluctuations.
>
> —Howard Odum, systems ecologist

THE ECOLOGICAL SYSTEMS APPROACH: VITAL FOR EFFECTIVE PREVENTION PROGRAMMING

A system is "a complex of elements in interaction, these interactions being of an ordered (non-random) nature" (von Bertalanffy, 1981, p. 109). In human development and psychology, an ecological systems approach places a person, often a child, in the center of progressively broader contextual influences and looks at the influences created by interactions among those systems. Research (e.g., Brounstein & Zweig, 1999) also shows that the most effective prevention strategies involve multiple systems. This ecological perspective suggests that programs need to address individuals as complex systems within other systems.

One systemic perspective is the ecological context model (Bronfenbrenner & Morris, 1998). The developing individual is embedded in several environmental systems pictured as ever broadening circles of influence. These settings surround the focal person and range from interactions with other people to societal or cultural belief systems. These ecological contexts have been organized into the following categories:

- **Microsystems** are the "inner circles," proximate niches, or "nests." These immediate settings include systems such as family, classroom, and neighborhood playgroups that most intimately affect the child.
- **Mesosystems** are the interconnections between contexts in which the person actively participates, such as partnerships between the family and school (for the child) or work spillover into the family (for the parent).
- **Exosystems** are settings that do not involve the developing person as an active participant but have an indirect influence. Examples are activities of the local school board, workplace policies affecting parental leave, and parent social support networks.
- **Macrosystems** are "overarching patterns of ideology and organization of social institutions" (Bronfenbrenner, 1979, p. 8) such as political, social, and cultural norms that lie further away from the individual.

All these systems interact, directly or indirectly, to shape development. Bronfenbrenner (1979) suggests that an individual's development is best served when there are strong supportive links between settings (family and school, neighborhood and larger community) and when the systems share common values regarding developmental outcomes.

In addition to these systems, time-related influences must also be considered. A person is not static, so past circumstances and the person's future orientation are important considerations when designing programs for youth. Strategies that consider the influence of time include:

- programs that are appropriate for developmental stages.
- effective timing of interventions activities. For example, programs for multi-problem, high-risk families have a greater chance to influence a child's outcomes if they occur early in the child's life (Bronfenbrenner & Morris, 1998; Cooley & Unger, 1991).
- components that help children to articulate positive visions of their future. Future orientation is a person's ability to project, set goals, and see a positive future. Children who have clear, positive future orientation are more resilient in the face of problems later in life (National Research Council, 1993; Nurmi, 1993).

Ecological and systems models permit valuable insights into the complex influences on developing individuals and draw attention to the ways individuals shape their own environments. These models also suggest novel and potentially powerful means of preventing later problem behaviors (Cowan et al., 1998; Schorr, 1989). In the sections following, we discuss systemic influences on development with an eye toward enhancing family functioning, as well as strengthening relations among children, families, and broader ecological contexts.

The Individual Viewed through a Systems Lens

Individuals are complex systems of attributes, response patterns, and genetic predispositions. These individual characteristics interact with and are shaped by external forces and experiences. The debate about which set of factors—nature or nurture—is the primary influence on developmental patterns has a long history (Plomin & McClearn, 1993). The interaction of these factors has important implications for any prevention or intervention program.

Prevention research also demonstrates that to understand later outcomes, one must consider both individual traits related to vulnerability and resiliency and the individual's experiences in the family and broader contexts. Numerous personal characteristics have been cited as increasing resiliency to substance abuse and other problem behaviors (Hawkins et al., 1992). Examples include academic success and social competency, autonomy, self-esteem, and positive social orientation (Garmezy, 1989), as well as the child's attributions about effort and ability (Rhodes & Jason, 1990). In addition to resiliency factors, risk factors also influence the individual. A review of research shows that multiple risk factors have more than an additive impact; they usually have a multiplicative effect on the individual (Coie et al., 1993). For example, an infant who has an irritable temperament is somewhat prone to be aggressive and antisocial in childhood. This risk can be magnified significantly when the child is reared in an authoritarian household (Coie & Dodge, 1998; Rutter, 1983b).

Practitioners who wish to implement effective intervention strategies must consider the multiple factors that comprise an individual's "person-system." Then, they must place those factors within the context appropriate for the individual, considering the various systems that affect and respond to the individual. Interventionists also need to increase their awareness of individual aptitudes or personality variables that might reduce responses to one form of intervention but enhance the benefits received from an alternative approach (Robertson & Reynolds, 1999; Shoham-Salomon & Hannah, 1991).

For the purpose of this monograph, microsystems are divided into family, peers, and the community, including schools. The macrosystems discussed are culture and society. The parent's social support system is a mesosystem (but part of the child's exosystem) that link the person with networks of extended family, colleagues in the workplace, and community professionals. We turn first to the latter setting, social networks.

CHAPTER 1

Social Support Networks Link Individuals with Ecological Systems

People's social networks reflect their individual characteristics and are influenced by features of the macrosystem. For instance, network composition is a product of one's cultural values and beliefs, ethnicity, income, gender, family structure, neighborhood and school environments, and personal values and beliefs (Cochran, Larner, Riley, Gunnarsson & Henderson, 1990; Cross, 1990). All of these variables motivate people to seek out certain types of social resources. They can also constrain their opportunities to do so. Conversely, influences from the macrosystem, in the form of cultural beliefs and practices or societal laws, may be filtered to the family through such social networks.

Networks provide both instrumental and emotional support (Belsky, 1984; Dunst & Trivette, 1990; Unger & Powell, 1980). Examples of instrumental support provided by social networks are material goods such as clothing and food, resources such as housing and transportation, and assistance such as advice, money, and child care. Emotional support would include respect, caring, and unconditional love. Social networks also involve social comparison processes ("Am I normal or atypical?"), social interaction, intellectual stimulation, feedback (including sanctions for behavior that deviates from norms or expectations), reflection of the self (Harter, 1999), socialization, role modeling, and stress buffering (Cochran et al., 1990).

Parents' support networks influence their child's development through direct interactions with the child but more often through influences on the parents. Emotional support often enhances parents' self-efficacy and reduces stress; instrumental support can include practical advice about effective child rearing (Cochran et al., 1990). A specific example is a study that looked at the relationships between social networks and parenting in different cultures. Regardless of cultural context or community setting (urban versus rural), parents who had more interconnected networks felt more competent. Also, more punitive parents had smaller networks, regardless of ethnic background (MacPhee, Fritz, & Miller-Heyl, 1996).

From a young age, children select their own social support networks, which include peers of about the same age and non-kin adults. Mentors, either adults or older peers, can be valuable additions to their networks, particularly as part of a program to improve school success and reduce problem behaviors (LoSciuto, Rajala, Townsend, & Taylor, 1996; Taylor & Dryfoos, 1999).

Prevention strategists can benefit from considering how relationships within one system affect relationships in other systems. For instance, children may behave differently with family members at home than with their teachers and peers in a day-care setting (Hinde, Tamplin, & Barrett, 1993). Also, the quality of the early parent-child relationship and social skills learned in the family context predict later peer relationships when the child enters school (Dishion, 1990; Ladd

& Golter, 1988). Such findings support the intervention strategy of developing family-school partnerships when targeting school achievement (Connors & Epstein, 1995) or problem behaviors (Bierman & Greenberg, 1996).

The Influences of Microsystems

Links between the Individual and Family Systems

A systems perspective involves examining how any stimulus or problem that affects an individual member of the family system influences every member of that family. Family systems theory (Cowan et al., 1998; Minuchin, 1985) asserts that the family's influence on developmental outcomes is based on complex, dynamic interactions among all members of the family, relationships among subgroups within the family (e.g., marital, sibling, parent-child), and a shared family history. Family members also bring their unique personalities into the equation, as well as their own perceptions of family dynamics, meaning that families *create* differences among their members (Dunn & Plomin, 1991).

Family factors are linked with future alcohol abuse and other adolescent problems. In a review of studies that followed youth from early childhood through adolescence, Zucker, Fitzgerald, and Moses (1995) identified several factors that are consistently related to troubled family dynamics and to problematic behavior at a young age. These factors include ineffective parenting; above average levels of parental psychopathology (particularly alcoholism); childhood antisocial behavior, aggression, and hyperactivity; early school problems; and poor peer relationships. It is interesting that these risk factors involve parent traits, child characteristics, and relationships within the family as well as with peers; that is, multiple systemic issues need to be addressed in prevention trials.

Programs can focus their efforts on different aspects of the family to prevent problem behaviors from emerging later. Although programs can be effective when they work with individual family members or with subgroups in the family, program benefits are maximized if both approaches are used in tandem (Cowan et al., 1998).

The first intervention approach focuses effort on individual family members. Because families operate as systems, changes in one member of the family should affect other members. For example, Gallagher (1990) noted that, "Teaching skills that make parents more competent also improve family interactions" (p. 543). Family members' feelings of powerlessness or their inability to use resources effectively have negative effects on the way they raise their children. Therefore, programs that empower parents can alter family dynamics in positive ways (Olds, 1997). However, interventions with just one family member are not always effective, even when they are as intense as weekly home visitor programs (Roberts, Wasik, Casto, & Ramey, 1991; Wasik, Ramey, Bryant, & Sparling, 1990).

Viewing the family as a functional whole is the contribution of family systems models, yet very few intervention efforts apply this concept. Typically, the individual parent is the focus of parent education efforts (see Cowan et al., 1998), or the individual child may be enrolled in an early education program to prevent school failure (e.g., Lazar & Darlington, 1982). Even when a more inclusive approach is taken, commonly one dyad such as the mother and child is the focus. Fathers, siblings, grandparents, and other caregivers play a secondary role if they are considered at all.

Parents and other family members who participate in programs that target only one individual, whether it is parent or child, often experience frustration and poor success when they return to their family unit and try to implement strategies or skills. At the very least, they often need to expend energy "educating" other family members (Nichols & Schwartz, 1995).

A second approach is to work with a significant portion of the family. Programs that target several family members and settings outside of the family tend to yield greater returns on the investment of intervention resources (Coie et al., 1993; Olds, Henderson, Tatelbaum, & Chamberlin, 1986; Schorr, 1989). When multiple members of the same family learn similar skills and share a common vision, the energy expended to create change within a household can be channeled toward the same goal. Interventions that focus on multiple family members affect both individual family members and relationships among them (Kumpfer & Alvarado, 1995; Miller-Heyl, MacPhee, & Fritz, 1998).

Research on substance use supports the wisdom of working with the whole family system. Both problem behavior theory (Jessor, Donovan, & Costa, 1991) and social–cognitive theory (Bandura, 1986) indicate that when family members do not approve of substance use, youth are less likely to experiment with drugs and alcohol (see Grover, 1998). Parents who carefully monitor their children's whereabouts, peer affiliations, and propensity for risk-taking have children who are less likely to experiment with substance use (Dishion, Reid, & Patterson, 1988). Conversely, when role models such as parents use alcohol or other substances and approve of their use, youth are at elevated risk for later substance abuse (Grover, 1998; Hawkins et al., 1992).

Family-centered approaches to preventing substance use are less likely to focus on the individual behaviors of children; instead, the trend is to focus on the family in a broader context (Grover, 1998). This trend acknowledges that families are connected to other microsystems and macrosystems to create a wide variety of developmental niches. A developmental niche is the physical and social context in which families and their children live, including their means of support, geographic location, and social networks with which they interact. These niches influence the family through prevailing child-rearing customs and parent attributes such as cultural belief systems (Super & Harkness, 1986).

The way parents react to their children in everyday life is linked with their experiences in these niches (Bronfenbrenner & Morris, 1998). Parenting reflects the economic situation in the family, the quality of day care and schools, neighborhood influences, other institutional organizations and social networks, and the wider social and cultural context. Consideration of the family system and the community context surrounding the family is important to developing an effective prevention program.

Peer Groups as a Microsystem

Parents and other significant adults play a central role in the development and socialization of children, but other children are also influential in the socialization process from an early age. The peer microsystem is important in helping children learn about themselves, as well as other people. Many competencies are best learned through interactions with others who are seen to be similar to the self (Hartup, 1989; Kupersmidt & Coie, 1990. Morison & Masten, 1991; Piaget, 1965). Peer interactions have important ramifications for social interaction, social perspective taking, and independent problem solving.

Piaget outlined how cognitive development, particularly in the area of moral reasoning, is influenced by interactions with peers who are perceived as social equals. These peers may operate on the child's level or slightly above. Social experiences with these equal-status peers result in problem-solving discussions that can broaden the child's perspective on an issue. Some discussions may lead the child to question the assumption that adult authorities have all of the answers, and other discussions may yield the insight that rules can be changed by social agreement.

Peer relationships are an important component of children's developmental pathways to later problem behaviors. Indeed, one controversial publication suggests that peers are much more significant than parents in determining developmental outcomes (Harris, 1998). Research does indicate that early social acceptance by peers is a key protective factor against later antisocial behavior (see Newcomb & Bagwell, 1996). Conversely, aggression leads to peer rejection (but affiliation with deviant peers), which in turn predicts later drug use, school problems, and criminality (Hawkins et al., 1992; Patterson et al., 1989; Patterson, Reid, & Dishion, 1992).

Peer cluster theory (Oetting & Beauvais, 1987) recognizes the influences of family, school, and religion on youth substance use, but adolescent peer groups are seen as particularly important. Peer clusters serve as a source of information exchange and value formation among its members. In this theory, the peer culture is seen as a direct causal link to adolescent drug use or a protective factor against it. This may be especially true if teens do not have close links with non-drug-using parents (Jessor et al., 1991). Research does support the presumption that affiliation with drug-using peers strongly predisposes youth, at least older ones, to use illicit substances (Brook, Brook, Gordon, Whiteman, & Cohen, 1986, 1990; Djazair, Donovan, & Costa, 1991).

Prevention programs must acknowledge the importance of the peer group in shaping attitudes toward and creating opportunities for risk-taking behavior in adolescence and then these programs need to create ways to expose youth to positive peer influences within a socially responsible context. Programs that involve group work with young adolescents do need to guard against deviant norms and behaviors that can develop as a result of the programs. For instance, some programs have found that young males will "one up" each other into using tobacco and alcohol, and the unintended consequence is that the intervention promoted the very behaviors it was supposed to prevent (Dishion, McCord, & Poulin, 1999). Programs also need to devise ways to foster youths' social skills, which should improve peer relationships, and teach assertive communication that would allow them to reject harmful activities in favor of healthy ones.

The School: A Microsystem with a Complex Influence

The educational system exerts its enduring influence on children from an early age, beginning in preschool, Head Start, or Even Start programs. School effects on academic and social skills and school-family partnerships continue from elementary school through college and beyond. Academic failure, especially in the late elementary grades, is a significant risk factor for later substance use (Hawkins et al., 1992), as are delinquency and association with deviant peers (Patterson et al., 1989). Further school dropout escalates these risks.

The influences of positive school environments are strikingly parallel to those of supportive family environments. And parents' connection with and support for the school contributes to their children's success in school. Some important parent-school connections occur when (a) parents value education and transmit that value clearly to their child, (b) parents monitor the child's behavior and performance at school, and (c) parents help their children to gain the skills they need to succeed in their academic tasks (Scott-Jones, 1995).

A school's overall environment influences individual children's adjustment and success. Battistich, Solomon, Watson, and Schaps (1997) showed that changing the school environment can significantly affect substance use and violent behavior. Schools vary in their climates and general expectations of all students (Bryk & Driscoll, 1988; Comer, 1980). The general climate affects both the teachers and the students in fundamental ways. Studies of "effective" and "ineffective" schools showed that children of all levels do better in effective schools (Rutter, 1983a). More dramatically, Rutter showed that over time, low achievers' academic success in "effective" schools was equal to high achievers' success in "ineffective" schools. In this study, neither the budget base, as long as it was above a minimal level, nor classroom size were significant determinants of effectiveness. Instead, the schools' social climate and values played key roles; an emphasis on academics, classroom management and discipline, and adult leadership made the difference (Rutter, 1990).

Like Rutter, Eccles (1993) observed that the better schools are marked by a confluence of sound management, emotional support, and high teacher involvement with and expectations of students. Children in such schools are more satisfied and motivated, may develop more autonomy, and have more positive self-concepts. They also capitalize more effectively on their individual strengths and preferences in classrooms where many activities occur, materials are varied in level and content, and they are given choice and control over what to work on and with whom.

Teachers contribute directly to students' academic and social successes within the school. Bandura's (1997) social–cognitive construct of collective efficacy (in the case of the teachers and staff of a school) explains why some schools are more effective than others in providing an environment where children can succeed. When the teachers and staff believe that, as a group, they have what is needed to ensure student success, the collective efficacy of those professionals will overcome the tight constrains faced by many schools.

Individual teaching self-efficacy (teachers' belief in their own ability to make a positive difference in the lives of their students) is important to creating successful classrooms. A teacher's efficacy beliefs influence the educational and personal outcomes of the children (Gibson & Dembo, 1984; Ashton & Webb, 1986; Greenwood, Olejnik, & Parkay, 1990; Fritz, Miller-Heyl, Kreutzer, & MacPhee, 1995). A teacher's sense of efficacy is one of the few attributes clearly linked with students' academic success in the classroom (Dembo & Gibson, 1985; Woolfolk & Hoy, 1990).

Both collective and teacher self-efficacy are key to children's success in school, but children's own self-regulatory processes are also central. Children's self-beliefs (appraisal of their own efficacy as learners) and the skills to monitor their own behavior determine children's school efforts and success (Zimmerman, 1995). Children's school experience and resulting sense of social and academic competence will shape their efforts and adaptability in later school years and adulthood.

In addition to academic instruction, schools provide a key socialization influence by teaching the community culture, directly and indirectly. The many years in school inevitably shape the personality and social behaviors of any child, as well as the academic knowledge and skills gained. The value of cooperative and competitive efforts, of persistence in the face of failure, of harmonious group relationships, or of individuality are differentially stressed in various cultural settings. Additionally, interactions with peers, teachers, and other families shape values and behaviors, particularly social skills. A teacher's response to a young child's conduct in the classroom or playground has been shown to shape the peer acceptance of the child (White & Kistner, 1992) and occasionally set up stereotype threats (Steele, 1997) for individuals that hinder both academic and social endeavors.

How might a systematic approach to prevention use this research on school effects? First, from the earliest years, programs should develop strategies to enhance a sense of purpose and support in schools, teachers' efficacy, and positive expectations of students. This should hold true whether it is at the preschool level or later. Second, research on family-school partnerships (see Connors & Epstein, 1995) suggests that programs would do well to increase family involvement in educational settings because both schools and families motivate, socialize, and educate children. Truly collaborative approaches encourage parents to shape the school's policies and practices and integrate families' knowledge, needs, and cultures into the life of the school. In a partnership-based model, school personnel may help families to develop their children's literacy, provide guidance on homework practices, and suggest ways to foster future college and career plans. Partnerships might also involve suggestions for effective discipline and guidance. Such partnerships would result in more consistent socialization in both systems, and lessons learned in one setting would be reinforced in others.

Culture and Community: Important Macrosystems

Social networks, families, schools, and peer groups are part of the larger culture that consists of particular beliefs and customs (Tietjen, 1994). Shared beliefs and customs influence and give meaning to the interactions that take place between individuals and their social networks. Therefore, supportive interactions may take different forms in different cultures (MacPhee et al., 1996).

These experiences, which vary across developmental niches, affect the types of competencies that children value and develop. The cultural macrosystem influences the specific competencies that children draw upon to interact with their particular ecological circumstances. For instance, in (Northern European, industrialized) societies where children are raised to establish their identities separate from their parents and to make their own way in the world, autonomy is valued and fostered (Harrison, Wilson, Pine, Chan, & Burie, 1990; LeVine, 1988; Triandis, 1995). In collectivist cultures, where conformity and obligation are valued, children are encouraged to stay close to the family. Education as a means of upward mobility may not be as strongly emphasized if it means leaving the local area (Caplan, Whitmore, & Choy, 1989; MacPhee et al., 1996).

Parenting strategies and the types of support structures around families also are influenced by culture. For instance, Native American families seem to be less punitive than Anglo families (Pettit, 1990; MacPhee et al., 1996). Hispanic parents who value conformity and obedience are more controlling and use harsh punishment more than other parents (Knight, Virdin, & Roosa, 1994; Quintana, 1991). African-American parents do tend to be more authoritarian, particularly in their use of physical punishment, but such practices seem to have adaptive value in keeping their children safe in dangerous environments. Authoritarian parenting does not consistently predict problem behavior later in childhood for African-American families, but it is a significant risk factor among Anglo families (Deater-Deckard et al., 1996).

An obvious implication of this research on cultural variations in child rearing is that prevention strategies are likely to be more effective when they are attuned to differences in values and beliefs, learning styles, and social networks. For instance, when social support systems involve much reliance on immediate and extended families, as in many Native American and Hispanic families, programs should consider involving multiple family members in an intervention program and provide activities for their involvement and learning. In cultures where parents may feel isolated or may not have much access to tangible assistance with child rearing, such as in some Anglo communities, programs may need to include concrete strategies for expanding parents' support systems. Disciplinary practices may need to be broached in culturally sensitive ways, too. Although spanking is a controversial issue in any group, being confrontational about punishment is likely to be counterproductive if parent authority and control are woven into the cultural fabric of parents' belief and traditions. Webster-Stratton and Herbert (1993) suggest ways that parent educators can sensitively address such strongly held beliefs.

A critical influence on families is their economic status and the general well-being of the neighborhood or community where they live. Low-income parents are more likely to be depressed, have poor self-appraisals, have more marital conflict, and use more punitive child-rearing practices (McLoyd, 1990). A comment by one of the mothers in our DTBY program poignantly captures these interrelated stressors: "No time. No money. I'm a frustrated mommy ... *I'm tired*." Similarly, deteriorating neighborhoods with weak social bonds tend to spawn child maltreatment (Garbarino & Sherman, 1980). Socioeconomic status is often viewed as an influence on families independent of their cultural background. However, the combination of economic and cultural constraints has a significant impact on the support systems that surround individuals and families. These structural forces in society limit access to networks because of group identity, access to social capital, economic limitations, and prejudice (Cochran et al., 1990).

Several studies that compare the effects of culture and socioeconomic status (SES) show that it is important to control for SES when comparing ethnic groups (Golding & Baezconde-Garbanati, 1990; Martinez, 1993). In a baseline study with participants in the DTBY program (MacPhee et al., 1996; Miller-Heyl et al., 1998), psychosocial risks accounted for many within-ethnicity variations. And when the differences in economic variables were taken into consideration, between-culture differences in important aspects of parenting disappeared. Stated differently, rural poor families of all ethnicities often had more in common with each other than more educated or more economically stable families from their own culture. One example of this was that poorer, less educated families were predisposed to use harsh punishment as a primary method for discipline. Therefore, prevention programs would do well to consider the economic status of the family, as well as the overall health of the community, when devising intervention strategies.

Mesosystems: The Connections among Systems

Considering the complexity of each ecological setting we have reviewed thus far, there are almost an infinite number of connections and relationships that could be developed among communities, families, and individuals. Instead of outlining all possibilities in this monograph, suffice it to say that programs are most effective when several of the systems that affect an individual are integrated in both the lessons taught and the strategies used in prevention. At least, strong prevention programs should work consciously to make multiple levels of the community aware of their philosophies and strategies (Steinberg, Darling, & Fletcher, 1995). When individuals hear the same prevention message from many sources, and their skills are supported at many levels, they are better able to implement new techniques.

We end this section on the systems approach with a general note of caution. The social integration of a neighborhood is important. However, even if a neighborhood is highly integrated and has many interconnections among supporting systems, children may not benefit unless their families also are socially integrated into the community. Perhaps day care centers, social services, health departments, and family advocacy services all work together to promote the same message about healthy families and positive behavior in youth. A community survey might rate a neighborhood as having strong connections. However, if a given family is alienated from these systems, the children in that family will not necessarily benefit from the intersystem connections.

KEY RESILIENCY FACTORS FOR INDIVIDUALS, FAMILIES, SCHOOLS, PEERS, AND COMMUNITY

The DTBY program is grounded in two theoretical perspectives: The ecological systems approach just covered and social–cognitive theory (Bandura, 1986) that deals with self-appraisals, attributions, problem solving, and relationship building. In this section, we discuss resiliency factors that are drawn from social–cognitive theory.

Efficacy Underlies Key Resiliency Factors

Self-efficacy is the perception that one can attain a given outcome or the belief that one can organize and execute actions required to reach a goal. For example, self-efficacy for a parent would be the belief that, "I can use a new parenting strategy effectively." It affects an individual's motivation to attempt new challenges and persist in attaining goals (Bandura, 1986). It is also strongly associated with a feeling of empowerment (Ozer & Bandura, 1990). People choose to act, or not, based on their efficacy beliefs (Bandura, 1997).

There is an important distinction between self-esteem and self-efficacy. Self-esteem relates to the way people feel about themselves in terms of global characteristics: I am a good athlete, I am intelligent, I am attractive, I can make friends. Such self-appraisals may be trait-specific, but they are not necessarily context-dependent. In contrast, self-efficacy beliefs are context specific. For example, a person's self-efficacy in public speaking will vary, depending on comfort with the subject matter and the perceived expectations of the audience.

Self-efficacy has many ramifications in a systems approach to prevention. Neither a child nor parent who has low self-efficacy will try new approaches to social interactions with others, and neither will they try new activities unless they believe that their efforts will produce positive results. People who have high self-efficacy in a situation will be motivated and persist in a given task, even when it is difficult.

Parent Self-Efficacy Relates to Skilled Child Rearing

Why should a substance abuse prevention program focus on parents' self-efficacy? First, parents of substance-abusing adolescents tend to be less confident (Rees & Wilborn, 1983), so low parent self-efficacy is a risk factor. Second, parents with low parenting efficacy will not try new disciplinary techniques or strive to improve their parenting strategies if they don't believe they can be successful. Thus, parent self-efficacy is an important mediator of effective child rearing, which in turn is a protective factor against children's substance use (Coombs & Landsverk, 1988; Holmes & Robins, 1988).

The premise that enhancing parental self-worth and parental self-efficacy can improve child rearing has been attacked by some critics who believe that programs to enhance individual self-esteem actually encourage narcissistic egocentrism at the expense of compassion and family health (Burr & Christensen, 1992). We do not share that opinion. Some correlational studies (Teti & Gelfand, 1991; for a review, see Teti, O'Connell, & Reiner, 1996) but not others (Brody, Flor, &

Gibson, 1999) find that mothers' self-efficacy beliefs correlate with child-rearing practices that promote children's competence. Additional research indicates that parents' well-being, in conjunction with their use of community resources, mediates the link between risk factors and nurturant parenting (Voydanoff & Donnelly, 1998).

Intervention studies clearly implicate parent self-efficacy as a mechanism of improved child rearing. For instance, Spoth, Redmond, Haggerty, & Ward (1995) found that maternal self-efficacy predicted changes in parenting skills due to a family intervention program, even after accounting for individual differences and program attendance. In the DTBY family program, changes in parents' self-confidence and efficacy also are strongly related to greater use of nurturing child-rearing practices (Miller-Heyl et al., 1998).

Confident Teachers Provide More Effective Learning Environments

In schools, teaching efficacy enhances the success of students (Woolfolk & Hoy, 1990). Studies of the process of teacher behavioral change indicate that staff development programs that focus only on knowledge and skills are ineffective. Programs need to enhance teachers' sense of support and efficacy. In fact, this should be done before introducing new materials. Enhanced perceptions of efficacy promote greater interest and commitment to implement teaching innovations (Greenwood et al., 1990; Woolfolk & Hoy, 1990). Teachers who have a high sense of efficacy tend to have classrooms that are warm and supportive. In turn, nurturing learning environments enhance learners' motivation and success (Bandura, 1986).

Therefore, when self-efficacy is strengthened, people are more likely to change maladaptive behavior patterns or learn difficult, new skills. In fact, we see improved self-efficacy as the key to effective intervention with parents, teachers, and community staff. A program that teaches parenting skills might do a very good job of providing information about effective strategies. However, if participants do not believe that they can effectively implement the new techniques, it is unlikely that those parents will actually try out their new skills. Time-out is a good example because it takes several weeks' persistence to implement effectively, and children's behavior typically gets worse before it gets better. As a result, many parents abandon the endeavor, especially if their confidence is shaky, and mistakenly believe that time-out is ineffective (Webster-Stratton, 1992).

Collective Efficacy is Important for Collectivist Cultures

"Collective efficacy" is another valuable concept. This occurs when a group, family, or community has a shared belief in its collective ability to produce outcomes. Collective efficacy is especially important when sociocentric cultures are involved. To collectivist cultures, the word "self-efficacy" may imply an egocentric concern with one's self-interest, which is anathema to the goal of working together to solve problems. People who work as a group instead of as individuals still must believe that together they can take the steps required to produce a desired result (Bandura, 1997).

To summarize, strategies that enhance and develop efficacy are essential to effective intervention programs. A primary step in programs should include the development of self-efficacy in peers, parents, teachers, or active community volunteers who will work with youth. When people in the social environment feel competent, youth also believe that they are capable.

Efficacy Supports Key Developmental Tasks in Children

Children's self-efficacy and social competence are key ingredients to successful adjustment. These resiliency factors are first acquired in the context of the family. Resiliency is enhanced when parents respond promptly and sensitively to the baby's needs (Finkelstein & Ramey, 1977), are nondirective but supportive, use "scaffolding" on problem-solving tasks (building on previous experiences and abilities), communicate acceptance rather than criticism, and provide mastery experiences that are moderately challenging (Bandura, 1986; Busch-Rossnagel, Knauf-Jensen, & DesRosiers, 1995). Research with the DTBY family classes shows that parents who perceive that they are competent are significantly more likely to use nurturing child-rearing practices (Miller-Heyl et al., 1998) and their children are more sophisticated in their ability to resolve interpersonal problems (Fritz, MacPhee, & Miller-Heyl, 1999).

The parents' ability to provide environments that enhance self-efficacy in their children is linked to many positive outcomes (Seligman, 1995). For instance, when mothers of Head Start children engage in educational activities at home, their children show higher levels of self-efficacy and better school adjustment (Mantzicopoulos, 1997). In longitudinal studies in which parents have been explicitly taught to foster children's curiosity, competence, and success, the children perform better on achievement tests and in school (Winter & McDonald, 1997). Both self-efficacy and school success protect children from problem behaviors such as substance abuse.

The school environment is also a crucial force in fostering children's self-efficacy. Several classic studies have demonstrated the effect of teacher expectations of performance on children's achievement and sense of competency (Rist, 1970; Weinstein, Marshall, Sharp & Botkin, 1987). Children's feelings of competency are basic to success within the classroom (Harter, 1983). A teacher who creates an efficacy-building environment can be a key source of support for a child. On the other hand, self-esteem, motivation, and coping can be adversely affected by failing to live up to the teacher's expectations (Connell & Ilardi, 1987). Efficacious teachers can provide environments that promote a sense of self-efficacy in children, and it is important that they do so.

Parents, teachers, and others who work with youth can learn and implement strategies that enhance children's efficacy, especially if adults believe that they are competent in working with youth. To summarize, all individuals, families, schools, and communities are affected by a range of social, economic, and cultural forces. Efficacious people are quick to take advantage of opportunities and can devise ways to overcome or avoid barriers.

The Role of Self-Esteem as a Resiliency Factor

As mentioned earlier, self-esteem has a meaning and role slightly different from self-efficacy. Self-esteem concerns children's global beliefs about themselves, particularly their self-worth (Harter, 1999). Although low self-esteem is a risk factor for later problem behaviors, high self-esteem does not guarantee protection against adverse outcomes. Such results have led to skepticism about the validity of boosting self-esteem as a prevention goal (Rutter, 1990). Others believe that self-esteem underlies the development of some key resiliency factors.

A close examination of these differing positions suggests that the disagreement is partly due to conceptual ambiguity. Some critics equate self-esteem with selfishness and egocentrism (Burr & Christensen, 1992), which obviously would not be a desirable outcome. Others say that strategies to boost self-esteem may lead to false or inflated self-appraisals, depending on how the program was implemented. However, most theorists define self-esteem in terms of global self-evaluations, whereas self-efficacy is one's judgment about competence within specific domains (Harter, 1992, 1999). These self-appraisals are based on one's sense of competence (self-evaluation), as well as the "reflected self," messages received from others in the social environment. It is important to note that competence is involved in both self-esteem and self-efficacy; the former is a *product* of perceived skill in a domain, whereas the latter involves a *motivation* to master or be competent. The motivational component is a core construct in DTBY because individuals who feel more competent persist longer at difficult tasks (Connell & Wellborn, 1991), and are more likely to engage in effective action (Markus, Cross, & Wurf, 1990). Poor self-appraisals, on the other hand, engender a sense of hopelessness about the ability to effect an action.

Therefore, programs that nurture self-appraisals must ensure that their goals and activities focus on developing the motivational component of competence as well as on accurate self-judgments. For example, the DTBY program for families does result in improved self-efficacy or competency beliefs, accurate appraisals, and persistence, but it is not necessarily designed to modify global beliefs about oneself.

Several Resiliency Factors Are Incorporated into Self-Responsibility

Self-responsibility is closely linked to and actually depends upon self-efficacy and self-esteem. As defined here, the acceptance of responsibility for making decisions helps a person reach chosen goals. It is influenced by

- self-appraisal of competencies,
- locus of control,
- attributions about the cause of past successes and failures,
- the sense of one's personal future, or future orientation, and
- the ability to identify feelings and effective responses in interpersonal conflicts.

Self-appraisals, which have already been discussed, are relevant because people are predisposed to take responsibility for actions when they have choices of which actions to take and when they believe that they can effect the necessary actions to attain a goal. Each of the remaining contributors to self-responsibility is discussed in later sections.

Locus of Control

In Rotter's (1966) classic work, locus of control involves people's global perception of how much control they have over outcomes in their life. People who have an internal locus of control believe that successes result from their own skill and effort and that failures are the product of insufficient skill and effort. In contrast, an external locus of control entails the belief that external factors primarily determine what happens in life, that one really has little influence over outcomes. Levenson (1974, 1981) distinguished between two forms of external control: a belief that powerful others control outcomes or that fate and chance determine what happens. We found the latter conceptualization appealing in our work because we thought that at-risk families, who may have extensive experience with the welfare and child protection systems, would have reason to think that "authorities" control their lives. The setting in which an individual lives does influence the balance of these two factors in a person's life. This concept is important to prevention because when people falsely believe that they have no potential influence over outcomes, even if they believe that they have the requisite skills, they tend to be apathetic and not take the action (Bandura, 1997). Conversely, if systems such as schools and community agencies are unresponsive to marginalized families' efforts to effect change, then it may be fruitless to convince individuals that they in fact control outcomes in those aspects of their lives.

Although both locus of control and self-efficacy beliefs are important to self-responsibility, they differ in important ways. Self-efficacy includes the belief that, "I can produce an action." Locus of control involves the consequence of such actions, summed across a range of endeavors: "In general, my actions have some impact upon what happens." Also, self-efficacy is specific to a particular outcome (it is context-dependent), whereas locus of control is a general trait. This latter distinction proved critical in our evaluations because DTBY produced reliable and large changes in parent self-efficacy but not in general locus of control. We believe that locus of control is more difficult to modify because it reflects lifelong experience in a wide range of contexts. Parents did report that they felt more "in control" of specific aspects of their family environment.

An interesting twist of locus of control theory is that prevention strategies might teach people to appraise situations with an eye toward creating positive changes in them. In effect, the onus would be shifted from individual accommodation or compensation for personal deficits (in terms of risk and resiliency factors) to modifying contexts. Such a strategy owes a debt to recent work in behavioral genetics, which suggests that people *seek out* experiences consistent with their genetic predispositions and *evoke* responses from environments that are consistent with these predispositions (Plomin, DeFries, & Loehlin, 1977). Some family therapists now help clients to identify ways in which their proclivities are incompatible with aspects of their environment (marriages, jobs), and then work on changing the context to fit the person better (Efran, Greene, & Gordon, 1998). Other examples include developing different or more positive social networks and encouraging parents to be more proactively involved in their children's schools.

Attributions about Success and Failure

Attribution theory (Weiner, 1986) describes how one's goal-oriented behavior is based upon the way a person interprets prior success and failure. There are two classifications of attributions: internal and external. Internal attributions about outcomes involve individual ability as well as the effort expended to achieve a goal (see Table 1.1), both of which are internal to a person. External attributions involve causes that are not under the person's control, such as the task difficulty and luck, either good or bad.

Attribution theory is a more complex variation of locus of control because the stability of internal and external attributions is considered. Thus, attributions to ability and task difficulty involve stable factors whereas attributions to effort and luck involve characteristics that vary across time, mood, and context. As such, people are likely to be more persistent, and their performance more predictable, when they believe that their success is due to ability (a stable factor) rather than their effort (an unstable factor). Although this theory has many implications for goal-oriented behavior, we focus on the importance of attributions to motivation. People are most likely to persist if they adopt a bias in which they attribute success to ability and failure to lack of effort, task difficulty, or bad luck.

Table 1.1.   Classification of Attributions
about Success and Failure[a]

	Internal Cause	External Cause
Stable Cause	Ability	Task Difficulty
Unstable Cause	Effort	Luck

[a]Adapted from Shaffer (2000).

We believe that attributions play an important role in mastery motivation and ultimately children's school and social competencies. As noted earlier, children are more likely to persist in difficult tasks if they believe that they have the ability but they just need to redouble their efforts. Conversely, children who attribute success to luck and failure to a lack of ability exhibit a pattern consistent with learned helplessness; they have "a cognitive set in which people believe that success and failure is independent of their own skilled actions" (Seligman, 1975, p. 38). They give up easily in the face of challenging tasks and are at risk for school failure and depression.

What experiences foster mastery motivation as opposed to learned helplessness? One influence is parents' and teachers' attributions for children's successes and failures (Dweck & Elliot, 1985), which are particularly evident in their praise and criticism. If children's abilities are praised when they succeed (as opposed to commenting on their hard work), it seems to motivate persistence. Children also tend to persevere in the face of failure when their lack of effort is noted. In contrast, their motivation will tend to be undermined by even well-intended criticism of their abilities such as, "This is hard for you to understand, let me help you." Why would one continue to struggle with a difficult task if one has been led to believe that the cause of failure is a lack of ability—an internal, stable trait?

Causal Attributions

Causal attributions have two implications that are relevant to this monograph. First, parent attributions about their children's problematic behavior are related to their anger and use of harsh punishment. Second, when youth make hostile attributions about a peer's (ambiguous) intentions, they are more likely to respond with aggression. Thus, contemporary intervention strategies that attempt to reduce hostile behavior in parents and their children often focus on the way they interpret social cues (Azar, 1997; Bierman & Greenberg, 1996).

Attributions are part of the schema that parents bring to the task of rearing children. Schemas shape interpretations of information that are encountered in any interpersonal situation. They are particularly relevant in interactions with young children, whose motivations often are not clear and must be inferred. As Azar (1997) and Bugental (1992) noted, the parent's own developmental history and personality can color these interpretive processes. For example, a parent who does not feel very capable or who is depressed might make a self-denigrating attribution about why her child misbehaved: "I should be able to control my child better, I must not be a very good parent." A parent who is rigid, has unrealistic expectations of children, or who operates from a threat-oriented belief system because of past abuse in relationships might make a child-blaming attribution: "My child is acting this way intentionally, just to make me mad." Or parents might attribute problematic behavior to either lack of effort on their part or to the difficulty in managing a situation (see Dix & Grusec, 1985): "Most children are tired at bedtime so her tantrum is pretty typical for kids this age, especially because I asked her to turn off the TV." Note that these attributional styles tend to reinforce parents' predominant schema.

Attributions appear to influence parents' child-rearing practices. First, abusive parents exhibit a negative attributional bias when they interpret their children's behavior (Larrance & Twentyman, 1983). Second, when parents make hostile or child-blaming attributions about their children's behavior, they become angrier and are more likely to select forceful, punitive strategies to gain compliance (Dix, Reinhold, & Zambarano, 1990; Dix, Ruble, & Zambarano, 1989). Parents also seem to take the child's level of competence into account. With older children, parents are more likely to infer that the child's deliberately committed misdeeds (when intention was ambiguous) and react with negative affect and power assertion rather than induction (Dix et al., 1989, 1990). Taken together, these results suggest that cognitive restructuring (Azar, 1997) may be an effective approach for parents who are predisposed to be angry and punitive in the face of fairly normal but stressful child behavior.

Such attributional processes also distinguish aggressive bullies from more socially skilled children (Dodge, 1986). In situations where a peer's intentions are ambiguous, children go through several steps in processing the social information available to them. Dodge (1986) has found that bullies tend to make hostile attributions in such situations. Further, such children are apt to prefer an aggressive response to more prosocial reactions such as information seeking. Bullies also underestimate the harm that their hostile responses inflict. (These processes are discussed more fully in the following section.) Not surprisingly, parents provide a rich training ground for these hostile social–cognitive processes. Parents who have hostile attributional tendencies use harsh punishment, and their children also generate more aggressive responses in interpersonal problem-solving tasks (Keane, Brown, & Crenshaw, 1990; Nix, Pinderhughes, Dodge, Bates, Pettit, & McFadyen-Ketchum, 1999). These children have more externalizing behavior problems and are likely to be rejected by their peers.

Decision-Making and Problem-Solving Skills Are Important to Resiliency

Once individuals believe that they can complete an action (self-efficacy) and that such action may make a difference (locus of control), they need to engage in decision making related to which action to take. We discuss two different resiliency factors that are related to decision making and problem solving. The first is a set of skills that include the abilities to (1) identify the problem or need for a decision, (2) think of alternative strategies, (3) predict the possible consequences of a given action (including the ability to take another's perspective), and (4) select an action. The second perspective on decision-making relates to the development of moral reasoning. This involves cognitive processes in which children engage when deciding whether an act is right or wrong (Shaffer, 1988, 2000).

Problem-Solving Skills as Resiliency Factors

Preschool and kindergarten children who can generate a number of alternative solutions to a problem and then assess the possible consequences of the alternatives show a higher level of social adjustment (Shure & Spivak, 1982; Shure, 1997). The ability to solve problems also has a positive influence on social adjustment and peer relationships in older youth (Haskett, 1990; Roopnarine, 1987), both of which are resiliency factors (Hawkins et al., 1992).

Children's previous experiences influence the way they apply their problem-solving skills. Children enter each social situation with a *memory store* of past experiences and a *goal*. For instance, the memory store contains past situations and the way the child has interpreted those situations, for example, "The last time I completed my homework, the teacher noticed I did a good job." The goal might be to make friends, have fun, or stay out of trouble (Crick & Dodge, 1994; Dodge, 1986). Dodge illustrated these processes with an example of a child who is tripped by a classmate while carrying a heavy load. First, the victim decodes the situation by searching for cues as to the reasons for being tripped, but notices only selected aspects of the classmate's actions. Second, the child interprets the action—by deciding whether the action was accidental, intentional, or ambiguous. These attributions will be guided by previous experiences with peers and in the family setting. Then the child thinks of possible actions and their consequences before responding. Although this is a simplification of the decision-making process, it points out that the child's interpretation of intent, as well as the child's social schema and knowledge, are primary factors in what action the child decides to take.

What role can families play in interpersonal problem-solving skills? As noted earlier, intrusive, controlling mothers tend to have children who are more disruptive and less competent in solving personal conflicts. Children who have problems in interacting successfully with peers often have authoritarian families, and the parents have low self-confidence, use praise infrequently, and exhibit poor parenting skills (Roopnarine, 1987). Poor relationships with parents are often duplicated in relationships with other adults or peers (Parke & Ladd, 1992). Abused children often have behavioral problems and poor problem-solving skills. They generate fewer and more aggressive solutions (Haskett, 1990). Given that the family is a training ground for poor or aggressive problem-solving skills, intervention programs need to enable parents to establish nurturing environments where positive social problem solving is modeled and encouraged.

Processes by which social skills can be transmitted from parent to child include modeling, discussing appropriate strategies, explicit coaching, and allowing children more latitude to make decisions (Parke & Ladd, 1992). Preschoolers who are successful problem solvers have parents who model or discuss effective problem-solving strategies that are geared to the child's cognitive level. This promotes more rapid skill acquisition (Pianta, Egeland, & Sroufe, 1990; Spivak & Shure, 1989). Parents' social cognitions also play a role in their ability to teach problem-solving skills. The mothers' causal attributions (see earlier section) are related to their anger and their disciplinary practices (Dix et al., 1990; Nix et al., 1999; Strassberg, 1995). Their beliefs play a role in the way they teach their children social skills (Rubin, Mills, & Rose-Krasnor, 1989). Aggressive parents can create an expectation in children such that they perceive the environment as hostile and believe that only aggressive responses will solve problems. This establishes an early belief system that predisposes children toward aggressive problem solving (Gabarino, 1992; Crick & Dodge, 1994).

Family disciplinary practices actually may have less influence on the child's interpersonal problem-solving skills than the parents' social cognitions, especially attributions that denigrate the child. Fritz et al. (1999) found that the way parents reason about social conflict is a model for their children for solving interpersonal conflicts.

A key risk factor for adolescent problem behaviors is aggressive behavior. Knowing that aggressive behavior is established early in development, it is obvious that intervention programs for at-risk youth need to help families and teachers modify the factors that contribute to antisocial behavior. Despite this widely recognized need, few programs focus on ways parents teach or foster their children's problem-solving skills (Bloomquist, August, Bromback, Anderson, & Skare, 1996). Prevention programs need to enhance parents' problem-solving skills as well as nonhostile causal attributions, nurturing parent practices, and the ability to notice and build upon the positive characteristics of their children.

The Health Belief Model

Decision-making skills also come into play when youth have the opportunity to engage in risk-taking behaviors such as drug use and unprotected sex. The importance of decision-making skills is illustrated by the fact that although many youth *know* more about AIDS and illicit substances after completing educational programs, their *behavior* often is not altered (e.g., Rotheram-Borus & Koopman, 1990; Slonim-Nevo, Ozawa, & Auslander, 1991). This led theorists and researchers to examine how youth assess risks to their health: how they reason about potential consequences, the importance of "personal fables" that lull one into believing that bad things happen to others but not oneself, and difficulties discerning causal links between behavior and high-cost outcomes. These aspects of reasoning improve with cognitive development, but early adolescence is a particularly vulnerable period because limited experience is combined with egocentric reasoning and more opportunities for risk-taking due to sexual maturation, availability of drugs, and access to cars.

Prevention programs that incorporate the Health Belief Model focus on personal perceptions of susceptibility to the negative consequences of high-risk behavior, the seriousness of these consequences, and the risk/benefit ratio of engaging in preventive behavior (Bush & Iannotti, 1985; Eisen, Zellman, & McAllister, 1985). For instance, perceived vulnerability is consistently related to abstinence from drugs as is the perceived seriousness of using drugs and overall concern for one's health (Kaufert, 1986). Individual characteristics also play a role in minimizing risk-taking behavior, particularly an internal locus of control and a positive self-concept (Bush & Iannotti, 1985; Hahn & Rado, 1996). Some intervention studies find that modifications of these cognitive risk factors do not necessarily result in long-term reductions in substance use (Ellickson, Bell, & McGuigan, 1993). However, we believe that teaching children decision-making skills, particularly consequential reasoning, has long-term benefit, so long as other resiliency factors are also fostered.

Development of Moral Reasoning

Most parents want their children to be helpful, caring, altruistic, and honest. Further, most parents hope that such behaviors are motivated by truly moral reasons—a concern for justice and the welfare of others—rather than self-interest or blind obedience. Therefore, parents should attend to their children's moral reasoning as well as actions. Programs designed to teach young children social skills or to prevent antisocial behavior will be most effective if they enhance youths' reasoning skills. For example, aggressive behavior is based on the intent to harm others, and it emerges as a stable characteristic early in childhood (Coie & Dodge, 1998; Eisenberg & Murphy, 1995). Combined, these two facts suggest that early intervention programs focused on preschoolers' social–cognitive skills, such as FAST Track (Bierman & Greenberg, 1996), should prevent later antisocial behavior. In this section, we discuss how children's reasoning, which depends on their cognitive development, changes predictably with age (Shaffer, 2000), and how socialization practices contribute to moral and prosocial development.

Piaget (1965) believed that moral development proceeds toward a respect for social rules and a sense of social justice. Although the concept of progression is still valid, it may actually occur earlier than originally believed. Current research has reevaluated Piaget's presumption that young children's decisions about right and wrong are based on an evaluation of outcomes or harm done, rather than intent or unquestioned acceptance of rules handed down by higher authority. More recent studies show that children as young as 3 to 5 years old distinguish between lies of deception versus misinformation (Siegal & Peterson, 1998). They also distinguish between harm that is the accidental product of good intentions as opposed to malevolence (Nelson, 1980). And they begin to recognize the social nature of rules. They can distinguish between rules that avoid harm to others versus social-conventional rules related to good manners or games. Violations of rules that result in harm are seen as more serious than violations of social rules, like breaking the rules in a game (Smetana, Schlagman, & Adams, 1993). Therefore, the groundwork for moral reasoning can begin with preschool-aged children.

Much of our understanding of moral development is based on Kohlberg's work (1976, 1984). He asked 10-, 13- and 16-year-old boys to resolve various moral dilemmas. Kohlberg was interested in the rationale that boys used to justify their decisions. He found that younger boys adhered to rules based on fear of punishment and the superior power of authorities. As adolescents are better able to take the perspective of other people and, eventually, the broader society, moral reasoning becomes increasingly more complex and concerned with universal principles of justice.

Kohlberg identified three levels of reasoning. In the stage of preconventional morality, youth conform to rules to obtain personal rewards or to. avoid punishment. Reasoning at this stage reflects self-interest and a dependence on authority. In the stage of conventional morality, which includes most adults, individuals obey rules to win approval for virtuous conduct or to maintain the social order. Obligation to law and order takes precedence over principled but "illegal" exceptions, such as civil disobedience. People who reason at the postconventional level have an internalized set of principles. They are committed to abstract, universal principles such as justice, individual rights, and the greater good. The goal of including activities in this area into a prevention program would be to set the foundation for youth to move out of the first stage into the second and third stages of reasoning.

People's level of reasoning is influenced by their experiences. Reasoning is not something that can be directly taught but gradually emerges from interactions with the social environment. Two processes are important in developing moral reasoning. First, interactions with individuals at a slightly higher stage than one's own may allow for insights into that level of reasoning. Second, cognitive conflict that challenges one's current mode of reasoning creates disequilibrium and may lead the individual to better understand a moral conflict (Eisenberg & Murphy,

1995). Either process may occur in the context of negotiation with others, group decision making or problem solving, and role-taking opportunities. For example, adolescents who are asked to discuss dilemmas and reach a consensus show greater increases in their reasoning, especially those who were lower than their peers before the discussions, compared to peers who made a decision without such discussion (Berkowitz & Gibbs, 1983).

How might parents promote more sophisticated moral reasoning and behavior? First, punishment is not likely to work because children tend to attribute their compliance with moral standards to external causes. (This enforces reasoning in level one, decisions made because of fear of punishment.) Instead, parents should combine expectations for compliance with methods that grant autonomy of choice. There are several strategies parents can use to encourage the internalization of values: (a) provide choices when making requests for compliance, (b) use suggestions rather than directives, (c) model a desired response instead of simply dictating it, (d) offer to share a task with the child, (e) emphasize the attractiveness of the desired activity, and (f) make statements that attribute the child's behavior to internal motives such as, "You are a helpful kid when you clean up your room" (Lepper, 1983). Note that several of these techniques require effective communication skills from the parent. Children's moral reasoning is also related to parenting styles that grant autonomy and to role-taking opportunities (Eisenberg & Murphy, 1995). For example, Socratic questioning, exposure to higher levels of reasoning, eliciting the child's opinion, and reflective listening promote moral reasoning whereas critiquing and directly challenging the child do not. Similarly, democratic disciplinary approaches such as induction and reasoning foster moral reasoning and prosocial behavior, but assertion of power does not.

Development of Empathy

Learning to feel empathy for the distress that one causes another person is a vital aspect of prosocial development. A lack of empathy is strongly linked with criminal behavior and violence, both in conduct-disordered youth (Coie & Dodge, 1998) and in adults with antisocial personality disorder (Marshall & Serin, 1997). We discuss it here because empathy is so clearly related to moral behavior, and it also is an integral part of social information processing. Children who are actively rejected by peers and adults because of their aggressive responses to provocation often underestimate the harm they inflict on their victims (Crick & Dodge, 1994).

Parents and others who work with children can use several strategies to encourage children to be empathetic. First, they can be good role models of empathetic behaviors by expressing sympathy for victims, showing distress when someone is harmed, and making reparations for harm done. Second, they can encourage children to attend to and accurately read cues that indicate how others feel. Finally, they can use disciplinary techniques that foster moral reasoning and moral behavior, particularly induction (victim-centered reasoning). However, when parents use punishment, children focus their anger and anxiety on the one who administers the punishment. This does not promote the development of empathy because it focuses children's attention, and often anger, on the person giving the punishment. A child believes that the uneasiness experienced is due to the punishment, an external attribution, not to the fact that they caused a problem for another person (Gilmartin, 1979; Turner & Finkelhor, 1996).

Rational, nonpunitive discipline such as induction promotes empathy by making children aware of the way their actions make others feel. Induction is particularly effective when combined with expressions of strong affect (Zahn-Waxler, Radke-Yarrow, & King, 1979) but not intense anger. The development of empathy is ineffective when parents rely on power-assertive approaches, such as, "You will do it because I said so." As children empathize with the victim and see that they are responsible for the victim's distress, they begin to make an internal attribution for their own uneasiness. They become less likely to repeat the prohibited conduct (Eisenberg & Fabes, 1998; Hoffman, 1984).

Induction, explanations of rules, and parent modeling of prosocial behavior all foster a concern for others, moral reasoning, and moral behavior. Why does such experience contribute to the ability to reason at a more mature level?

- The explanation for the reason why a behavior is problematic provides standards or rules that children can use to evaluate their actions.
- Stressing the needs and emotions of others encourages the development of empathy and reciprocal role taking, two cognitive abilities that facilitate mature reasoning.
- Induction allows parents to talk about the affective components of ethical development, noticing clues about the feelings of others.
- Parents can use this as an opportunity to explain what the child should have done and what the child can now do to make amends for the transgression.

Therefore, induction is an effective method of socialization because it demonstrates the effective, cognitive, and behavioral components of ethical development and may help the child to integrate this information. The focus on the child's thoughts and feelings rather than the imposition of external control promotes the kind of attributions that contribute to internalized standards and self-regulated behavior (Eisenberg & Murphy, 1995).

Parent–Child Communication is a Key Resiliency Factor

Parent–child communication is related to a host of outcomes in adolescence. When parents have an open style of communication with their teens (Kafka &

London, 1991), are skilled at conflict resolution (Hops, Tildesley, Lichtenstein, Ary, & Sherman, 1990), and express their values about health and risk-taking (Reis, 1996), their adolescents are less likely to use drugs. On the other hand, when parents express less positive regard, are inattentive listeners, and deny feelings, their teens are at greater risk for problem drinking (Jones & Houts, 1992). Similarly, delinquency is less prevalent in families characterized by open communication and skilled problem solving (Clark & Shields, 1997; Klein, Forehand, Armistead, & Long, 1997). And positive peer relations are correlated with open communication and involvement of the child in collaborative decision-making in the home (Fuligni & Eccles, 1993; Hinde & Tamplin, 1983).

Why might family communication play such an important role in promoting positive outcomes in youth? At least three processes might be implicated. First, parents who are skilled in resolving interpersonal conflicts in the family are modeling, if not directly teaching their children, strategies that can be employed with peers (Parke & Ladd, 1992). This social learning process is likely to have a direct effect on peer status and social competence, which in turn protects against antisocial behavior and drug use in adolescence (Patterson et al., 1989).

Second, open communication is consistently related to youths' feelings of self-worth or self-esteem (Demo, Small, & Savin-Williams, 1987; Jackson, Bijstra, Oostra, & Bosma, 1998; Stafford & Bayer, 1993). The affective tenor of open communication seems to be particularly important. Burnett (1996) found that the frequency of positive versus negative statements was more strongly related to children's self-esteem than the parents' own levels of self-esteem. When parents convey approval and acceptance—unconditional positive regard—it enhances their children's sense of self-worth or self-esteem (for reviews, see Feiring & Taska, 1996; Harter, 1999), and this acceptance is typically communicated with I-messages rather than blaming and contempt. In multi-problem families, bad feelings result from failures to listen nonjudgmentally to each other and from active criticism. Poor communication skills in such families predisposes parents to rely upon coercion and physical discipline to influence children's behavior (see Blechman, 1991).

A number of prominent parent education programs teach parents how to convey acceptance through I-messages and reflective listening. These programs include Systematic Training for Effective Parenting (Dinkmeyer & McKay, 1976) as well as *How to talk so kids will listen & listen so kids will talk* (Faber & Mazlish, 1980). I-messages "own" the parent's feelings and focus on the misdeed without denigrating or labeling the child. Reflective listening or "checking out" acknowledges the child's feelings and perceptions and helps to match the intended message to its impact on the listener (Blechman, 1991). (Keep in mind the fact that recent, rigorous research by Gottman and colleagues [1998], on predictors of divorce and marital satisfaction suggest that the regulation of negative affect is highly important.)

Many parent education programs also teach parents how to explore alternatives and collaborate in problem solving to minimize blame and anger. Examples of approaches to family problem solving include the family meeting, no-lose conflict resolution, and leaving notes (see Faber & Mazlish, 1980). The common thread among these techniques is that they establish a climate of trust and mutual respect, attend to problem ownership, and develop children's self-worth.

Third, the message's content instructs children about rules, social norms, and standards of behavior. When parents use induction ("How would you feel if …?") after the child has harmed another, it not only induces empathy for the victim, it endorses the Golden Rule (Zahn-Waxler et al., 1979). When parents clearly convey their values about substance use and early sex, their children are less likely to engage in deviant or risky behavior, so long as the parents are not coercive and are role models of responsible behavior (Hahn & Rado, 1996; Reis, 1996). More generally, clear communication about rule violations and parent expectations, when combined with follow through (i.e., consequences rather than empty threats), socializes children to have a moral compass and to regulate their own behavior (Baumrind, 1996).

In sum, research on parent–child communication illustrates its functions within the family: to exchange information and increase understanding, to develop rapport and trust, to problem solve and resolve conflicts, and to transmit emotion (Kieren & Doherty-Poirier, 1993). Communication also is the means by which family members continually negotiate or define the nature of their relationships (Watzlawick, Beavin, & Jackson, 1967). Parent-to-child communication is particularly likely to involve behavior management: requests (versus coercion), approval (versus criticism), and rule statements (Blechman, 1991). All of these processes are fundamental to the family's well-being, which is why so many parent education programs, marital enrichment curricula, and family therapy frameworks focus on communication skills. Notably, few programs work with the whole family (Cowan et al., 1998; Kieren & Doherty-Poirier, 1993). The DTBY curriculum does have the traditional emphasis on effective communication, but it incorporates innovative, age-appropriate strategies that can be used by preschoolers and parents alike.

Ecological Systems and Social–Cognitive Development Theory Applied to Early Prevention Programming

The DTBY program for families who have 2- to 5-year-old youth is a practical application of ecological theory to early prevention programming. This is done through a series of classes that involve preschoolers and multiple members of the family. Preschool educators and community members who work with families are also involved through DTBY school and community training. By including these additional systems, the effects of intervention on the families are reinforced and maintained.

Family and community classes focus on developing children's social–cognitive skills. The curriculum is also designed to build resiliency to adverse circumstances, such as deviant peers and denigrating messages from others, and to reduce risk factors. This chapter describes how each element of the program translates the theoretical concepts discussed earlier into effective practice.

APPLYING SYSTEMS THEORY

As discussed in Chapter 1, the more congruence and interaction among systems, the more potential effect there will be on individuals. The DTBY program illustrates the multiple level approach that includes the individual child, family relationships, expanded support systems, and the community context. Intervention strategies directed at each of these levels are discussed in the sections that follow.

The main focus of this monograph is on the program for families of preschoolers, although as shown in Chapters 3–5, other components focus on school, community, and peer contexts.

The Individual Child Is Directly Involved

A special program is designed for preschool participants. Attributes that confer resiliency are fostered in developmentally appropriate ways. Upon entry into the program, adult and teen educators work as a team with the youth for 10 to 12 weeks, two hours per week. The child-to-staff ratio is approximately one teen or adult for every three to five preschoolers. Trained "Teen Angels," who work under adult supervision, are assigned as the constant companions of three to five preschoolers for the duration of the program. This low ratio ensures individualized and nurturing relationships for each child. The children's program runs concurrently with the parent program.

The Family System Is Involved

All family members are encouraged to participate because when more than one caregiver is involved, family-based programs are more effective. Caregivers may include the father, mother, grandparents, stepparents, and extended family who have primary caregiving roles in the child's life. This approach is so important that an incentive package is used to recruit multiple adult family members into the program and to keep them involved for the entire program. This incentive includes family meals, a nonjudgmental environment, fun, and upon completion of 20 hours of the program, a $200 honorarium for each fully participating adult family member. There was a 95% retention rate in the initial program, and 45% of the families included the father's participation.

Brothers and sisters also have a significant role in the family. They are encouraged to attend the workshops and participate in a corresponding curriculum designed for 6- to 12-year-old children. Each night of the program might go something like this: After a social time and family dinner, family members participate in classes that are divided by age group but still have a common theme for the evening. The age groups usually include 2- to 5-year-old children, 6- to 8-year-old children, 9- to 12-year-old children, and the parents. Youth who are 13 and older may become Teen Angels who work with the younger children.

Time is set aside at each session for special parent–child joint activities that involve the focal preschooler. This gives the families structured time to enjoy each other while reinforcing a key learning goal. Usually, the activity is congruent with the daily theme. For example, if the topic for the session involves identifying feelings as part of improved communication or empathy development, the parent–

child activity might be the "feelings cube." A large cube has a face on each side showing six different feelings. Parents and children take turns rolling the feeling cube and then describe a circumstance when they experienced the indicated feeling, for example "I was scared when ..." or "I was happy when ...." This simple activity reinforces empathy development and permits the members of family groups to practice communication skills with each other.

Support Systems Are Enhanced

Adult family members have an opportunity to expand or strengthen their support systems. Sometimes participants need to strengthen relationships within the family, if they are frayed, but others might want to expand the number of non-kin relationships in their network. (Research on personal social networks shows that adults tend to turn to different resources to meet particular needs, such as child care, financial help, a sympathetic ear to talk about family issues, or employment contacts [Belsky, 1984; Cochran et al., 1990; Unger & Powell, 1980]). The program approach provides opportunities for the parents to strengthen relationships with both kin and acquaintances. For example, support systems are enhanced through the social time and family meal that begins each session. Staff members sit with different families at different meals. Arranged seating with place cards can be used to encourage families to intermingle so that they get to know each other.

Other program features that promote social support include norm setting (where the group establishes norms governing their conduct in the classes), small group activities, normalizing of difficult parenting situations, and a nonjudgmental environment. Webster-Stratton and Herbert (1993) discuss how essential these approaches are to the impact of parent education. Not surprisingly, DTBY participants are significantly more satisfied with their support networks after completing the workshop series. On open-ended questions that ask about the best part of the workshops, participants also usually list normalizing parenting problems and enhanced support systems among their three favorite features of DTBY.

Effective Programs Maintain Continuity of Interactions with the Family

Initially, the families participate in a 10- to 12-week series of classes. Including the meal and the parent-child joint activity, each class lasts 2½ hours. Classes are best scheduled so that the entire series lasts three to four months. At the end of each series, continued support is available through two mechanisms. Yearly reinforcing workshops are scheduled as boosters for the families. These booster programs have four classes that support and expand upon the original concept. As in the first series, all family members are encouraged to attend. Meals, the children's educational program, and a financial incentive of $50 per adult are offered.

Periodic support groups, called AFTER-DARE, are offered in addition to the reinforcing workshops. In some communities, alternative family activities such as "Winter Games" (described later in this chapter) are preferred. Participation in AFTER-DARE is entirely elective, and no financial incentive is provided.

Peer Support Systems Are Developed

DTBY incorporates positive peer influence on the children through both the teen teachers and the positive environment of the youth classes. The Teen Angels (trained teen educators) provide positive role models and peer pressure for positive behaviors. In many cases, these teens actually take the role of mentors with the younger children. The small teacher-to-student ratio enhances the nurturing environment. The individual attention and program activities allow children to develop relationships with other youths their age in an effective "alternative activity." Mutual support, fun, and learning occur. Parents are present and indirectly involved, and the families are connected to each other through a common activity (class participation).

Training for Teachers Includes the School System

For 2- to 5-year-old children, the school environment is their preschool, Head Start, or other early education or day-care program. As discussed earlier, teachers and the school environment exert an important influence on the development of youth. To involve this system, special workshops were designed for the preschool, Head Start, or day-care providers who were involved with children in the program. These were adapted to meet the needs of the different community environments. Two of the original sites were actually sponsored through Head Start/day-care facilities. The staff training and activities provided by the DTBY program became a key element in their staff development and philosophy. Thus, the youth experienced DTBY precepts in two settings. In addition, the home and school environments had a strong, compatible philosophical connection through the program. In other sites, day-care providers and other preschool teachers were specifically targeted if they worked with the families in the program. Although this is a looser connection because the entire preschool was not usually involved, it still provided the additional connection to the school system.

Community Team Training Adds More Interconnections

Community team training is an integral piece of the multilevel intervention. Agencies that work with youth or their families are invited to participate in a 15-hour community facilitator/team training. This training is founded on the same principles as the family and school training (see Chapter 5 for content) but is adapted for wider use by community agencies or volunteers. To optimize its effectiveness, a minimum of six agencies or organizations should be involved. It helps to develop a common philosophical base and terminology among the systems. It is also designed to strengthen the personal efficacy of the participants in their work with families or individual youth and to provide strategies to enhance their existing youth work. Our approach involves some strategies that are incorporated into community asset building (Kretzmann & McKnight, 1993), although there is less emphasis on organizing grassroots efforts by citizens to identify resources in the community.

Cultural and Socioeconomic Macrosystems are Considered

DTBY was implemented in a wide variety of cultural and socioeconomic settings. This required a program model that could be adapted to varied needs and that would value strengths inherent in diverse groups. Program sites were encouraged to hire staff who were culturally competent and accepted by local families. Staff training focused on the key content variables and processes and also on adaptations that would be relevant in that particular setting. If we think of developing resiliency in youth as the ultimate destination, our process consists of defining key landmarks (training objectives) and suggesting several routes (activities and strategies), but the individual site teams determined the actual course. This travel plan might include a side trip to include culturally relevant information.

Another important element is to help families discover the strengths inherent in their culture and community, so that they can build on these resources. One example of the way this happens is a parent–child activity where the family builds a paper representation of their home, an origami house, a paper tepee, or a hogan, and decorates the home with pictures that show family members strengths or values.

Given that families from different cultures may have unique needs, it is important that the program offer multiple options for activities. An example is the After-DARE support groups and community activities. In the original study, young, single, and predominately Anglo mothers preferred a regular support

group where they could get together for educational or recreational events and
have their children in a corresponding program. They needed the expanded circle
of friends. In the more collectivist communities where there was more family
involvement, families did not desire a regular support group but preferred family
events where they did activities with each other and their children. An instance of
this was an event we called Winter Games. This event was held in a local dining
hall that was turned into a winter playland with fake snow (huge bags of shredded
paper from the local newspaper). Families enjoyed fake skiing, sledding, building
igloos, and many other "winter sports." The educational objective was to share
ways to have fun with children inside during the winter (although we didn't
recommend filling their homes with shredded paper!).

SOCIAL–COGNITIVE THEORY GUIDES
THE PROMOTION OF RESILIENCY AND RISK
REDUCTION

Many resiliency factors are linked with positive youth development. Often
prevention programs try to promote one specific factor, or "magic bullet." However, a combination of factors produces the best results. The review of social–
cognitive theory in Chapter 1 suggests that fostering self-efficacy ("I can implement an action") is only the first intervention step. A larger effect will occur if
people develop self-efficacy plus an internal locus of control ("If I take an action,
it may have the desired effect"), as well as problem-solving strategies ("Among
my alternatives, this action may be the most effective in the long term"). Thus,
several skills and beliefs are needed to actually produce the results.

Research in the prevention field tends to treat each of these factors separately;
that is, self-appraisals, locus of control, and problem solving. This has led to
mixed reviews as to how important each construct, considered *independently*, is
for later outcomes. Yet Bandura's social–cognitive theory asserts that all three
components are necessary to children's social and cognitive abilities. Therefore,
effective programming needs to include all three steps. The foundation for all
three cognitive constructs must be laid early in life, even for children who do not
yet fully grasp cause and effect reasoning. In DTBY, self-appraisals, locus of
control, accurate attributions, and problem-solving skills are combined into a
unified curriculum. Children who participated in the program showed a significant
increase in their developmental level over control peers, which may indicate that
the combination of the three is indeed effective. Higher scores on developmental
surveys in preschool children indicates a greater school readiness. In turn, school
readiness is linked with school success and attachment to school, which are well-
documented resiliency factors.

Strategies to Enhance Efficacy Beliefs and Self-Esteem

When people have a strong sense of self-efficacy or believe that they will succeed in important endeavors, they are more likely to try new, potentially difficult tasks and to persist in completing these tasks. One strategy for building self-efficacy is used weekly with both children and adult family members in the family classes. In an activity called Success Sharing, the definition of success is expanded from having money, possessions, and status to include the everyday accomplishments that a person completes just to get through the day. People are asked to tell about small successes they had during the week. This may be as simple as getting the laundry done or staying calm in a stressful situation. This process of accentuating the positive encourages family members to look for their accomplishments instead of focusing on their failures. It is especially important that this activity is repeated weekly so that participants get into the practice of noticing small successes during the week.

Expectations for the classroom environment are established for both adults and children to provide mutual support and a nonjudgmental atmosphere. These expectations are conveyed in part by staff and in part through mutually agreed upon class rules (see Webster-Stratton & Herbert, 1993). Collectively, the classroom process and repeated activities are designed to help people identify their strengths and develop self-efficacy.

Many of the activities for parents include group discussions that implicitly normalize the difficulty parents have with their children. These discussions also illuminate a variety of parenting options in difficult situations. Thus, parent classes focus on both expanding the parents' self-efficacy and giving the parents skills to expand the self-efficacy of their children.

Many of the activities for children actually build competencies. At snack time, the children may learn to pour juice and make no-bake cookies. In other activities, the children may produce new types of artwork or learn new songs.

Development of Self-Responsibility Is a Major Component

As outlined in Chapter 1, this construct includes four components in addition to self-efficacy. These are internal locus of control, accurate attributions about the causes for success and failure, future orientation, and the ability to identify feelings and effective responses in interpersonal conflicts. Because of the wide range of cognitive development of the participants, from preschool to adults, each of these processes is modified with a variety of strategies and activities.

In preschool-age children, the classroom management style establishes a pattern for internal control. For instance, puppet skits depict several choices of behaviors that children may choose in the classroom. Some are appropriate (sharing), and some are not (hitting). Children vote on whether they want to have that behavior in the classroom by voting either "thumbs up" or "thumbs down." This strategy empowers them to set the "rules." The puppets also demonstrate the consequences of making a choice that violates the classroom rules. In most cases, it is a gentle time-out. Then, when children choose an unacceptable behavior, they are reminded that they made that choice. Staff members also are attentive to "good" choices and acknowledge them.

Locus of control is fostered by having the preschoolers tell of situations when they used their "personal power" in positive ways (good choices) or in ways that were not so good (poor choices). This personal power activity is also an effective parent–child activity and adult activity. For adults, perceptions of control are modified in activities that have them consider times when they say, "I have to...." This activity helps parents to see that often they have actually made a choice for very good reasons, yet they were unconsciously attributing their actions to some undefined external source.

Parents also learn how different behavior management strategies help children to internalize social rules. Thus, parents are taught strategies that set clearly defined limits with input from the child, as in no-lose conflict resolution. They are encouraged to allow choices within the framework of the limits and to provide consequences when these limits are violated. Consistent with the literature on communication, parents are taught effective problem-solving strategies to resolve conflicts. Strategies that develop empathy or role taking are also discussed because they encourage children to learn self-control and are a foundation for good peer skills, as well as moral behavior.

Self-responsibility also includes attributions about the cause of past successes and failures. In the children's program, teachers explicitly comment on the children's abilities and skills when they are successful; when a child fails, teachers attribute it to the difficulty of the task or lack of effort. Through modeling and instruction, parents also are taught how to attribute successes to ability rather than to effort or luck. These strategies keep families motivated and also enhance self-efficacy. Parent attributions also play a role in the way they interpret their children's behavior, so we help parents to understand the reasons for their children's misbehavior. When children act out, punitive or coercive responses tend to create child blame or self-blame because such methods lead children to be angry and resentful rather than to focus on the problematic behavior. When parents have a more realistic idea of what to expect from children at different stages or that a problem might be situational rather than a deliberate provocation, they may be calmer when dealing with the child's behavior. Role-taking skits, in which parents experience being "children," help them to understand children's behavior in difficult situations and increase empathy.

Future orientation is a person's vision of that person's future. As an early component of the classes, adult family members are asked to set a personal goal to achieve by the end of the class and another to achieve in one year. They are also asked what they would like to see developed in their child by the end of the class and in one year. (This activity also helps families to articulate their values and motives.) This task was surprisingly difficult for most participants, which emphasizes the importance of formal activities that encourage such visioning.

The ability to identify feelings is a precursor to managing behavior and making personal choices. Awareness of emotions and communication skills are woven into all aspects of the program. Activities range from the "feelings cube" described earlier to skill building for recognition of feelings in adult family members. The staff models the skill of acknowledging feelings and encourages development of a feelings vocabulary throughout the program.

The ability to identify multiple possibilities for responses to interpersonal conflict is incorporated into the self-responsibility activities described earlier, as well as into the decision-making component of the curriculum (see following).

Families Learn Decision-Making and Problem-Solving Skills

There are several skills that are traditionally linked with problem solving. These include the ability to define a problem, the ability to think of numerous choices and their potential outcomes in a situation (which also includes evaluating risks), and the ability to prioritize. Strategies and activities to develop these skills are built into each age level of the program. A sample activity in the parent curriculum is the "Control Auction." This activity has many educational objectives including prioritization of different aspects of one's life over which a person would like to keep a sense of internal or personal control. This process of prioritizing builds decision-making skills.

One of the steps in problem solving is to evaluate the consequences of behavioral choices. Ideally, this evaluation is informed by judgments about the rightness or wrongness of actions, which relates directly to moral reasoning. Moral reasoning is grounded in a developmental process where children internalize principles that help them to distinguish between right and wrong and then act on the distinction (Eisenberg & Murphy, 1995). Only when children internalize positive social standards will they act responsibly outside the presence of an authority figure. Moral development includes feelings one has about a decision or behavior (the affective component), the ability to inhibit harmful actions such as lying and stealing (the behavioral component), and the child's (or adult's!) decision about whether an act is right or wrong (the thinking component).

The feeling component has been addressed in the self-responsibility section of this chapter. Preschoolers can start to manage their behavior (behavioral component) if they have models, such as puppet skits, and consistent management strategies used by adult caregivers. The use of inductive discipline strategies in the children's program promotes empathy, so that children understand their impact on others. As discussed in Chapter 1, children as young as 3 years old begin to recognize the nature of rules and can distinguish between rules to prevent harm to others and "conventional" rules, like rules in a game (Siegal & Peterson, 1998). For the thinking component, the preschool activities include only a few rules and build on the skills of identifying feelings and making simple choices. Children also have input into the rules set for the classroom. Puppets act out various behaviors that children might exhibit in a classroom, like sharing, hitting, and climbing. The youngsters get to vote (thumbs up or thumbs down) on which actions they believe belong in a classroom. A chart reminds them of what they have decided.

There are a number of activities and educational materials for the siblings and adult family members that support this construct. Part of the curriculum for adult family members includes a discussion of Kohlberg's (1984) theory of moral development. This provides a basic level of knowledge that is often missing in parents. Many of the activities cover ways to identify feelings, manage their own behavior through stress management strategies, expand the number of choices they have in situations, and determine consequences for choices. Parents are exposed to management styles that promote decision-making and problem-solving skills in their children, such as induction and reasoning. They are also taught methods to develop problem-solving and conflict-management skills in their children. The process of the classes helps family members learn decision-making skills by turning problem solving back to the participants.

Social and Communication Skills Are Included in the Curriculum

Isolation and antisocial behavior are high-risk predictors of problem behaviors in youth. In contrast, the ability to establish healthy relationships with a wide variety of people is a resiliency factor, as is the ability to resist negative peer pressure. These processes of building support and resisting social pressure involve assertive communication and other social skills. Not incidentally, these same skills also promote positive family relationships.

The DTBY curriculum reinforces social skill development at all ages. Role-taking activities are minimized before the age of five because young children have a limited ability to make clear distinctions between their own and others' points of view. Activities with preschoolers focus on reinforcing socially appropriate behaviors and modeling social skills. Some coaching occurs to facilitate social skills.

Puppet skits show how aggressive dinosaurs who have no friends can learn to be less aggressive, use positive friendship skills, and make friends. Puppet stories also show how dinosaurs can move from playing alone to playing with other friends. Preschoolers can practice the different skills in role play using puppets. In the class, the staff encourages cooperative work and games that involve all of the children.

Perspective-taking and role-taking activities receive more emphasis in the classes for parents and older children. Empathy development is a central goal of these exercises. From third grade on, children's ability to see the other person's point of view, their role-taking ability, has been shown to influence their peer group status (Kurdek, 1982). Therefore, activities that show how another person is feeling are an important part of the curriculum from early childhood through adulthood. Activities for adults focus on basic communication strategies such as reflective listening; understanding the differences between aggressive, assertive, and submissive behaviors; and ways to select the appropriate communication strategy in different situations. The skills are built around communications within the family and with social support networks outside of the family.

3

DARE to be You Children's Program

The DTBY program for children consists of three mutually supporting aspects: a broad spectrum of educational activities for the youth; strategies for the parent, teacher, or other community member to use with youth; and environmental structures to enable the participants to learn and practice the desired skills. The curriculum includes a preschool activity book (for children 2½ to 5 years old), a curriculum volume for children in grades K–2, a volume for grades 3–5, and a volume for grades 6–8. These include developmentally appropriate activities for each age group. The materials can be used with just one age group or in consecutive years because activities for older groups build upon those for younger children. The curriculum may be used in the children's component of a family program (as described in this monograph) or in a school, after-school program, community, or church-based youth group or camps.

High school age students have their own curriculum. Although the activity manual for this age can be used with teens as the focus of intervention, the DTBY philosophy is to involve teens as teachers or program aides in the community. Therefore, the teen or peer curriculum is designed to train adolescents to work with other youth in the community. For example, in the program for families of preschool youth described in this monograph, teens are trained to work with the younger children in the program.

DEVELOPMENT OF THE CHILDREN'S COMPONENT

The children's component began in 1979 with a focus on 8- to 12-year-old youth. The original project was developed and tested through the 4-H youth

41

program of Colorado State University. The development team included health education specialists, teens, parents, teachers, and 4-H club leaders and agents. The Centers for Disease Control (Risk Reduction Initiative) funded research on the impact of the program. Experimental and control groups were randomly selected from schools and 4-H clubs in Weld County, Colorado. A two-year follow-up showed significant differences between the two groups in the onset of use of alcohol and tobacco, as well as in communication and decision-making skills (Miller[-Heyl], 1981).

Then, the program was offered to numerous communities in Colorado and other states through community team training. Participants in community team training were contacted for annual follow-up surveys. Feedback from these surveys consistently pointed to a need for an expanded version that could be used with youth from kindergarten through high school. Funding from the U.S. Department of Education in 1982 allowed development of the K–12 Substance Abuse Prevention Curriculum. This three-year research project included field testing the new curriculum in control and experimental schools. The results included a significant increase in teacher efficacy in the experimental group compared to the control group (Fritz et al., 1995).

Follow-up surveys with community team members also identified the need for programs for families, especially families with young children. Again, this was congruent with the ecological theory underlying the DTBY program. Funding for the development of the program for families was provided by the Centers for Substance Abuse Prevention in a 1989 High Risk Youth Demonstration Grant. This original demonstration grant was implemented at four diverse sites in Colorado to determine its effectiveness with a variety of cultures: a Native American site in southwest Colorado; an urban site in Colorado Springs; a rural, traditional Hispanic and Anglo site in the San Luis Valley; and Montezuma County, a rural and multiethnic site in Southwest Colorado.

As described in Chapter 6, the children's developmental levels showed statistically significant improvement. The program was subsequently replicated in other sites and with other target populations: through the Asian Association of Salt Lake City (Utah) with six Asian and Pacific Islander populations, a Hispanic and an Anglo population; in California with African-American and Hispanic populations; and in Colorado in a small urban community (Pueblo), with several rural Navajo communities in the southwest, and with Head Start populations in southwest Colorado.

PROGRAM FOR 2- TO 5-YEAR-OLD CHILDREN

Although the activities for preschool children can be used in any setting, they were specifically designed for use in conjunction with a simultaneous parent program in the family component. For example, when the parents are involved in the self-efficacy/self-esteem section of workshops, the children also have activities on self-efficacy/self-esteem. Similarly, preschoolers, older children, and the parents learn about effective communication (e.g., "Thumbs Up") in tandem.

The children's program benefits from a low student-to-teacher ratio. For every four to five preschoolers, there is one trained adult or teen teacher. The program always has a trained preschool program coordinator. This person oversees a team of trained teen helpers (Teen Angels) who are assigned as constant companions to the children throughout the course of the 10- to 12-week series of workshops. Although the teens could be volunteers, experience has shown that a paid teen staff provides the necessary consistency and quality.

An important part of the children's program is the parent–child activity that occurs in each session. This lasts approximately 15 minutes and is designed with the attention span of preschool children in mind. It revolves around the same educational objective for the session that guides activities in the parents' and children's groups.

The curriculum activities are designed to teach the social–cognitive skills discussed in Chapter 2. The complete set of activities for preschool-aged children may be found in the DTBY Activity Manual for Preschool Youth and in the Parent–Child Activity Manual available from the authors. Activities that support each of these resiliency factors are discussed in separate sections that follow.

Self-Esteem/Self-Efficacy

Activities for preschoolers revolve around building competencies and recognizing strengths and positive characteristics. A parent–child activity that exemplifies this process is the "Complete Child." In this activity, parents trace their children on large pieces of newsprint or heavy brown wrapping paper. The parents and children work together to think of positive characteristics or abilities that the child has. They illustrate the tracing of the child with pictures or words that identify those characteristics. Characteristics must be seen as positive and valued by the parent, and they must be honest. If a child is not a fast runner, that should not be listed. Parents are encouraged to be very specific and to have "proof" of characteristics that they share with the child such as specific occasions when the child showed the ability or trait. To end the activity, family groups take turns standing in front of the group and showing their drawings. This gives children the opportunity to hear their parents describe their positive features to others, much like Faber and Mazlish's (1980) strategy of letting children hear the parent say something positive about them.

Other activities occur in a "Circle Time" that involves only the children and their teachers. Children may take turns telling about some ability or characteristic that they have, such as "I can tie my shoes," or "I help my mommy." This helps children learn positive self-appraisals.

The staff members consciously make attributions that encourage internally motivated behavior and self-appraisals. They do so with comments on natural abilities or acquired skills when the child is successful, but they attribute failures to lack of effort, difficulty of the task, or other attributes that are unstable or external to the child. The positive attributions follow an important format. Rather than a very generic "good job," staff are encouraged to identify a "powerful word" that describes a characteristic and then "give the proof" or describe the event that proves that person has the characteristic. If the staff notices that a child often helps, such as picking up art supplies the staff member dropped, and they want the child to see herself as helpful, the staff member would say, "You are a helpful person. Look at how you helped me pick up all of these markers."

Activities to encourage positive self-appraisals also involve learning skills to cope with events and circumstances that can undermine self-esteem. Some activities help children value differences in themselves and others; others help children learn ways to deal with negative comments ("killer messages") from other people. A self-efficacy or self-esteem activity is included in every class meeting.

Activities for Self-Responsibility

Preschool children can begin to understand that their actions have effects. DTBY integrates this concept in an activity called "King and Queen of Hearts." Children take turns being the king or the queen. At their "coronation," they receive a crown and a scepter (wand). They get to select an action they would like the rest of the class to do such as act like a bunny or butterfly, hop on one foot, or dance. They wave their wand, which "causes" the teachers and other classmates to all act like bunnies until the child waves her wand to stop. Preschool children very often do not have an experience of this type that so clearly illustrates how a choice they make influences the actions of others.

Another series of activities helps preschoolers learn to expand their vocabulary of feeling words. Staff members enhance the children's ability to recognize feelings through classroom strategies. The "Bearometer" is a chart that is mounted on the wall with a picture of a happy bear on one end of the chart and an unhappy bear on the other end. When children arrive at the program, they are encouraged to color their own bear, draw in the mouth showing how they feel that day, and tape it to the wall. This gives the staff an opportunity to recognize and validate the child's feelings before the class starts.

The concept of personal power is reinforced with "personal power stars." Children color and cut out large stars that are illustrated with pictures of situations in which they used their "personal power" to make good choices such as to do something that was helpful or kind.

Classroom strategies also contribute to enhancing self-responsibility. Puppet plays that allow children to participate in voting on classroom rules and the use of inductive or intrinsic classroom management styles lay a foundation for developing a sense of responsibility. Allowing children to be responsible for some aspect of the program, like setting out the snack or pouring juice, also gives them a sense that they can complete a task and that it will make a difference.

Techniques designed to help young children learn stress and anger management are included. Children learn that feelings of stress and anger are normal but it is important to be able to direct anger in ways that do not harm others. Children learn a song, "Use a word," to remind them to use words when they are upset rather than hitting another person. They also are allowed to "pound playdough" as a stress management strategy. Although this activity is offered as a regular option in the children's class, it is also used as a special parent–child activity.

Decision Making and Problem Solving

Many of the preschool activities affect various developmental concepts that are core to the program. Having input into class rules, as described previously, influences decision-making skills because it helps young people to internalize the social norms of the classroom. By using their thumbs to vote on what behaviors they want in the classroom and which ones they do not want, they have concretely contributed to and "bought in" to behavioral norms.

Each class includes time for optional activities; the children can choose which one they want to do from a menu. Book reading can also develop decision-making skills when the teacher uses dialogic techniques (Whitehurst, Arnold, Epstein, & Angell, 1994) such as, "How does she feel when her friend teases her?" and, "What do you think she should do next?"

Teachers encourage children to solve problems by having them come up with several choices they have in a situation. These steps are familiar to readers who know negotiation or conflict-resolution strategies: identify the problem, encourage ideas where both children in the situation can have their needs meet, have the children think of five possible solutions and what might happen if they chose those actions, and make a choice. This process requires staff time, which is one reason that a high teacher-to-student ratio is important to the program. Although this strategy may not be employed in each situation where a problem arises, it is important that it is applied part of the time. The message sent to the children is very powerful: You are capable of solving this problem, you can think of many good ways to handle situations, and you do not always need to depend on others to tell you how to act. This approach thus encourages internalization of rules and social problem-solving strategies.

To emphasize the importance of including this strategy, consider what would happen if a child always depended on adults to intercede. The message is equally powerful when someone else solves one's problems or "rescues": You are not capable of solving problems, someone else has to give you ideas, and you need to depend on others to know how to act. When children consistently have their problems solved for them, they are trained to have an external locus of control and to attribute their success to luck or situational factors.

Empathy is developed when the staff uses the simple strategy of having one child look at another to see if each can discern cues as to how that child is feeling. This is done in happy situations and in conflict situations. In another activity, "Sharing Sarah," the child program coordinator brings a treasured old toy to class and tells the history of the doll or toy and how important the toy is to them. This nurtures the sense that adults have feelings much like those of children. Then the children are allowed to gently help take care of the treasure. The "Feelings Cube" activity, described in Chapter 2, gives the preschoolers a forum to talk about situations when they were scared, happy, or sad. Thus, the other children hear that others have similar feelings, which also normalizes such reactions to situations.

Social and Communication Skills

Stories and puppet plays are important means of teaching social and communication skills to preschoolers. One story tells about a dinosaur that has trouble making friends because she is very aggressive and the other dinosaurs do not want to play with her. The children come up with ideas that the dinosaur might try. The mother dinosaur also gives the children "tips" for making friends. This method gives children vicarious practice with friendship skills to see what the consequences of different strategies might be. Other stories show the differences among passive, aggressive, and acceptable (assertive) behaviors so that children can see acceptable behavior modeled. Children are involved by coloring different characters and acting out the story.

Some activities help children learn listening skills. For instance, children are given a picture of a dressed-up elephant. The teacher reads a story and they fill in colors and parts of the elephant that match the story. The importance of listening is reinforced visually as the children see their elephant completed.

EARLY CHILDHOOD CURRICULUM

In the family program, this curriculum is used with the siblings who are 6 to 8 years old. This curriculum can also provide important life-skills training in classrooms, after-school programs, or in other youth groups. It follows the same social–cognitive developmental model as the preschool curriculum. A complete set of activities may be found in the DTBY School Curriculum, Volume II for grades K–2.

The group structure and management strategies are important. Independent decision-making is promoted by allowing the youth to contribute to the rules and norms of the group, by providing choices, and by using induction and reasoning.

As with the preschool program, the staff focuses on positive behaviors and strengths. The activities are designed to appeal to a range of learning styles.

The curriculum is designed to be used in several ways. A series of up to 20 activities can be used in each grade level. These can be used with just one grade level or in consecutive years to build upon skills learned in previous years. After-school programs can use the curriculum to add a life-skills component to other activities. Community youth groups can use it to develop leadership skills in young participants. Camps can incorporate the curriculum into other activities.

Self-Efficacy/Self-Esteem

At this age, children begin to notice the attributes of others. One of the activities that encourages children to notice and value others is "Smile Circle." Children cut out big circles with smiles printed on them to hand to their neighbors in the circle. They are to tell their neighbors one characteristic that they like about them. The comments, which vary with developmental level, might range from "I like you because you are friendly" to "You draw really pretty pictures."

"I'm Taking a Trip" is an activity that is effective in valuing differences, especially with second graders. One child sits on a chair in the center of the group, pretending to be in a one-person spaceship. The only way that she can take her trip is if she can find something that is different about herself from everyone else in the class. The most effective way to start is with a characteristic that is so inclusive, it includes most of the children in the class—such as "I like to play in the water." Then all of the children who like to play in the water gather around the spaceship. The person on the "ship" continues to add skills or experiences that are true for her. If other children have not had that experience or do not have that attribute, they sit down. Once children sit down, they have to stay down—the criteria are cumulative. The final goal is to be the only person left on the spaceship so it can take off. The child on the "spaceship" usually has to think hard to find something special and unique about herself that is different from everyone else in the class. This is a fun way for children to identify their unique attributes and also to learn to value differences. The child who begins with a broad category such as "play in the water" may end with a list that includes a memorable boat trip or a special swimming skill she has.

Self-Responsibility

Activities at this age level continue to build skills in recognizing feelings. For instance, "Stand Up" begins with a description of different situations in which children might find themselves. A series of flash cards with pictures of faces that illustrate different feelings are held up. Children stand up when they see the card that portrays the way they would feel in that situation.

At this age, children begin to internalize appropriate behavior in relationships. One activity to support this ability involves having children describe actions they might take that would influence whether or not they would make or keep a friend. The children brainstorm actions they could take that build friendships and other kinds of actions that might harm friendship. In this way, their repertoire of strategies is expanded, and they learn more about the consequences of their behavior with peers.

Puppet shows, stories, and role modeling are especially powerful at this age. "Dyna and her friends" describes a well-intentioned tyrannosaurus whose group-entry skills leave a bit to be desired, and so she alienates potential friends in her new neighborhood. As the story is told, the children are asked why Dyna's playmates didn't want to hang around her, and what might be more effective ways to make friends than to barge into a play group.

Decision-Making, Communication, and Social Skills and Substance Abuse Awareness

These components build on the theoretical base outlined in Chapters 1 and 2 and again include developmentally appropriate activities. In kindergarten, children identify people that influence their decisions. They are encouraged to become aware of the effects of their actions on others. Related to communication skills, they learn ways to say, "I don't want to" in potentially dangerous or harmful situations. Activities primarily involve storytelling, puppet skits, and role play. First and second graders learn to read others' body language through group activities. They learn skills to make and refuse requests through assertive behaviors. Three dinosaurs behave in ways that mirror their names and illustrate aggressive, passive, and assertive communication strategies: Greedy Grabby Gertrude, Wishy Washy Wilber, and Ask Nicely Annie. These dinos all teach children that particular social skills, or their absence, affect relationships with peers and are more or less effective in problem-solving situations.

CURRICULUM FOR MIDDLE AND LATE CHILDHOOD (GRADES 3–5)

Developmental goals are slightly different for this age group from those for the younger children. This is reflected in the curriculum. Although many activities continue to build on skills and insights that were introduced with the younger age groups, activities are also expanded to include new concepts. The peer group becomes more central in children's lives, so that some activities help participants to consider different aspects of friendship. For example, the activity "Friends, how they help, how they hurt" normalizes the challenges of relationships and provides ways to cope with and benefit from friendship issues. (DTBY School Curriculum, Volume III for grades 3–5).

The self-responsibility section includes practical applications such as time management and responsibility for wise choices during free time. Children also can become aware of the power they give others over their actions and feelings and learn strategies to maintain internal control.

Communication activities help children become aware of ambiguous or double messages and what to do about them. Consistent with the research on attributions and peer skills, children are taught to ask clarifying questions and accept compliments. Resistance strategies are introduced in this age group.

In the decision-making segments, priority setting, goal setting, and determining choices and outcomes are introduced. Students practice reasoning skills in role plays. Students also become aware of roles people take in social situations. An example of this is creating a "family mobile" that shows how something that affects one member of the family also influences the other members.

CURRICULUM FOR EARLY ADOLESCENCE (GRADES 6–8)

Early adolescence is a time of rapid social and cognitive change. Youth face multiple challenges and can expand their competencies very rapidly at this age. Activities for this group continue to build upon previous skills. However, they also specifically address issues that are especially important in the middle school years. (DTBY School Curriculum, Volume IV for grades 6–8.)

Future orientation becomes more important as youth begin to explore their identities. One activity encourages youth to project a positive vision for themselves in the future. The stresses in early adolescence can seem overwhelming. Self-efficacy activities at this stage help the young adolescents recognize that they have the capacity to deal with problems. One activity, "Stormy Weather," increases awareness of problems they have already solved or tough times they have already "survived" to give them a sense of capability in this area. Body image and concepts of adulthood are the topic of several activities.

Activities for self-responsibility expand to include ideas of group dynamics, self-defeating behaviors, and motivations. They also identify areas in which youth should maintain control of their behaviors instead of giving "control" to friends. Two strategies develop this concept. A ROBOT Worksheet has youth think of "buttons" that they allow others to push. Some of these buttons, when pushed, might lead to decisions that are not in a person's best interest. They identify the buttons that they will not let others push. Another strategy is an activity called

Strings that is described in Chapter 4. This activity allows the participants to see a visual representation of times people give control of their actions and feelings to other persons. A clear distinction is drawn between positive strings (parts of relationships that enhance a person's well-being) and negative strings (the aspects of relationships that can harm a person).

Decision-making activities include strategies to help youth see others' perspectives. Many activities in this age group build on cognitive dissonance, such as the game "Agree/Disagree." In this activity, participants stand on either side of the room according to whether they agree or disagree with a controversial statement made by the facilitator. Then, they have opportunities to share their conflicting viewpoints on the issues in a controlled debate. The end point is not so much "winning" but whether or not the participants have expanded their ability to see different views of an issue. When students are queried about the activity later, their responses usually indicate that the majority of students now have broader views of the issue. This format capitalizes on the increasing ability of adolescents to see multiple perspectives.

The curriculum also helps youth learn and practice more positive communication strategies such as assertiveness and peer-resistance skills. Positive family communication is emphasized, as youth become better able to take others' perspectives including the perspective of their parents.

PROGRAM COMPONENT FOR LATE ADOLESCENCE (PEER CURRICULUM)

As stated earlier, the DTBY philosophy is that teens, especially in late adolescence, are resources in their community. This also fits with the social and cognitive developmental stages of older adolescents. They are beginning to see themselves as members of larger society, and taking social perspective is important at this stage. They are also an incredible resource in the community in their role as peer leaders, helpers, and educators. They often have the energy and passion for making changes. They have budding leadership skills that can be directed in positive ways. (DTBY School Curriculum, Volume V, Peer Leader's Manual.)

Therefore, the curriculum for teens takes a capacity-building approach. Teens who participate in the 25 class periods outlined in the curriculum are introduced to the theoretical foundation of DTBY, experience activities to increase personal efficacy, learn interpersonal helping skills for peers, and learn to lead activities and workshops to improve life skills. After the students complete the curriculum, they may use the information personally in peer-helper relationships; in mentoring, cross-age teaching, leadership for school and community projects;

and in community educational projects. Camp counselors find that this curriculum is a useful tool for training junior counselors.

In the DTBY program for families with 2- to 5-year-old youth, the peer curriculum provides the foundation for training the Teen Angels in the program. In the DTBY family program for juvenile diversion, this curriculum guides the activities that are employed with both adolescents and adults taking the classes.

An example of an activity in this curriculum is the "Time Line of Responsibility." Teens are given 3 × 5 cards, each with a description of a different behavior or responsibility. A long piece of butcher paper that has sections for ages ranging from infancy through adulthood, including a "never" category, is spread on the floor. Teens decide at what age youth should be able to begin the different behaviors, such as having certain chores, dating without a chaperone, taking a paid job, first kiss, and many more. Teens place their cards (anonymously) face down on the time line at the age that they believe is appropriate for starting the behavior. The cards are turned up and the age-appropriateness of that behavior is discussed. The person who placed the card can choose to defend its placement or not. Then, teens repeat this procedure from the perspective of a younger brother or sister, or they can project themselves into their future role as a parent. This tool helps to expand the perspective-taking abilities of the participants and also opens the discussion to many issues around self-responsibility.

Even though teens are an important community resource in working with other youth, there are pitfalls to consider. Teens must always be under the supervision of an adult who can guide them without being coercive and controlling. Adolescents often believe that they can go into a setting and facilitate one of the activities because the materials and instructions seem simple. However, without preparation and practice, conducting activities that build life skills can be much more difficult than they seem. A perceived failure on the first attempt can be very disheartening. Adults who work with teen helpers or mentors must establish mechanisms that permit teens time to gain supervised practice and enter their work prepared.

Classroom management skills take time to develop and are not easily mastered. The most effective approach pairs a group of teens with an adult who is skilled at classroom management and facilitation; this adult oversees the teens and gradually shares more of the responsibility for the class. Debriefing sessions after programs or classes are an essential aspect of highlighting emergent skills and providing feedback. Programs that use teen mentors or teachers can cause more harm than good if careful supervision, constant support, and opportunities to practice are neglected. "Pep rallies" to boost the teen workers or volunteers are also important. Working with youth can be exhilarating but also exhausting and discouraging. Pep rallies help teens on a team celebrate their accomplishments.

4

DARE to be You Family Program

The family curriculum evolved from our work with community teams because these community partners also perceived a pressing need for early prevention strategies that involved collaboration with families. Also, there is a natural fit between DTBY's theoretical foundation and work with families. Both social–cognitive theory and the ecological systems perspective emphasize the importance of processes that develop within the family, as well as connections among multiple systems.

The more family members who are involved in a program, the greater the chance that positive changes will occur in that family. Therefore, the program is designed to include more than one adult family member. Mothers, fathers or father figures, grandparents, aunts, and uncles are examples of key family members who may play a primary role in rearing child. All are encouraged to attend. Preschool children may be the focus of the program but siblings are included and have their own special curriculum. The recruitment and retention incentives are a key to enticing families to participate and retaining them throughout the entire program.

RECRUITMENT OF TARGET POPULATION

The program has been replicated in a wide range of urban and rural target populations, as well as different ethnic groups. Recruitment strategies have varied with cultural and community context. However, a few factors seem to be consistently important across diverse circumstances. First, the more agencies and organizations that are involved in the initial planning stages or are involved in DTBY community training, the broader the base of support. A community collaboration can cast a wide net when recruiting families. Second, the people who recruit for the program are the first contact with the family. These people must be able to model the nonjudgmental DTBY philosophy, emphasize strengths, and empower families.

Third, recruitment and screening efforts should be mindful of optimal class composition. In the original high-risk youth trial, families were recruited to fit a risk profile. No more than 10% of the families could have more than seven of the risk factors (see Table 4.1), approximately 80% of the families had two to seven risk factors, and 10% of the families had fewer than two risk factors.

This profile has several advantages and fits the theoretical base of the program in a variety of ways. First, the potential stigma attached to attending parenting classes is reduced if the program incorporates at least some families who are perceived to be healthy and functioning well. When all participants are "high risk," it is easy for the community to equate DTBY with fixing pathology or remediating problems. Second, the effectiveness of the DTBY process is compromised. For example, one strategy is to move people from one level of reasoning to a broader or more advanced perspective. This approach requires that some of the people in the group actually do reason at a higher level. Much of the class process involves problem solving and role modeling around child management issues, and so the parents need to be exposed to a range of strategies that might work with

Table 4.1.   DARE to Be You Risk Factor Index

Risk criterion	Pretest variables
Maltreatment	1+ foster-care or shelter-home placement in last year
	Prior mandated parenting classes
	High use of harsh punishment (Disciplinary Practices Report)
School failure	Mother's education < 12 years
	Father's education < 12 years
Economic disadvantage	Annual family income < $15,000
	Unemployed wage earner (parent)
	Welfare (AFDC, tribal allowance, food stamps)
	Assistance from employment agency in last six months
Mental health issues	Individual or family therapy in last six months
	Community agency help with individual family problems
History of substance abuse	Immediate family had/has problem with alcohol or drugs
	Spouse history (as above)
	A.A. or Alanon in last six months
Situational/developmental	Teen parent (now < 20, or < 24 and first birth < 20 years)
	Socially isolated (Social Network Questionnaire)
	Foster parent
Community risk	More than 80% of families have substance abuse problems
Violence	History of violence or delinquency
Long-term health issues	

their children. Finally, a varied risk profile in class is an asset in building support systems and normalizing parenting problems.

Class size is important to consider. The optimum size for the adult component of the class is 12 to 25 adults. Although the program still is effective when enrollment deviates from this range, the activities are designed for groups of this size. Because the entire family is invited, the number of children often is a key consideration. In communities where family sizes are small, 25 adults may bring only 13 children. In communities where family sizes are large, 15 family units might translate to 60 children. The number of staff members who are available determines how many children can participate and still ensure a quality experience. The facility is also important because it must be accessible to the families (travel distance is an issue in rural sites), able to accommodate groups of children as well as the parent classes, and be user-friendly in terms of climate and the ability to conduct educational activities.

RETENTION STRATEGIES

One of the biggest frustrations for organizations that conduct parent classes is that once families are recruited (not an easy task itself!), it can be quite difficult to get them to attend all of the classes. Agencies often expend significant resources organizing and holding a series of parent classes, only to have poor registration and attendance rates. When this happens, there is little or inconsistent impact (e.g., Resnick, 1985) and the resources are wasted. Therefore, retention strategies are critical to the ultimate success of a program.

The incentives for the DTBY program include these four strategies:

- Family meals are provided at each session. Free food always is an effective inducement, as long as it is of at least modest quality, but family meals also provide a low-stress means to meet other families and to ease into the evening's work.
- The program has a family focus rather than a parent focus. The entire family is invited to attend. Children are not simply in child care; they are enrolled in an educational class. (Some parents do not come for themselves; they come because the children enjoy it so much.)
- A warm, nonjudgmental environment where people feel supported and their strengths are recognized. The fact that parents learn valuable skills and their children like the program also helps.
- Often the most controversial incentive is a $200 honorarium for each adult family member who attends at least 20 hours of the parent classes and parent/child activities. Adult family members must sign in at the time they

arrive and sign out when the leave. The staff is responsible for noting if participants leave early. Individuals who have poor attendance are required to forfeit the incentive or attend make-up sessions.

The incentives encourage male involvement: 45% of the family units in the original trial included fathers, stepfathers, or grandfathers. It also recruits families that might not otherwise participate. Retention across sites—families who complete all of the classes with their children—averaged between 90% and 97%, which is quite high considering the risk status of many participants.

FAMILY CLASS LOGISTICS

The optimum format is a series of 10 to 12 workshops scheduled weekly over a period of three to four months. Each of these workshops includes a family meal/social time (about 30 minutes), a parent–child activity (approximately 15 minutes), and then separate classes for the adults and the children. The children's classes are described in Chapter 3. These classes are 1¾ to 2 hours in length. The total time per session is approximately 2½ hours; families do not get "credit" for the mealtime. Any evaluation activities involving completion of baseline and posttest surveys are in addition to the 20 to 26 hours of classroom time. In the pilot year of the parent/preschool program, one facilitator provided the entire curriculum as an intensive weekend seminar. Although the total number of contact hours with the families was similar to the usual 10- to 12-week format, there was no discernible impact on participants. It is essential to introduce ideas and strategies over time, so that new skills are practiced and assimilated as a foundation for later activities.

The facility can influence the effectiveness of the program. Space should include a place to prepare and serve a meal, and means to clean up and put away the food before the program starts. One workshop space needs to be large enough to accommodate both parents and their focal preschool child for the parent–child activity. This may double as a parent classroom or as one of the classrooms for the children. The ideal facility has a playground and four workshop spaces for parents, preschoolers, infants, and older siblings.

STAFF TRAINING

Trainers and Coordinators

The staff in the family program is structured as a team. Therefore, parent trainers and child program coordinators are trained together even though the components for the adults and children differ developmentally. This co-training allows mutual understanding of the educational goals of the parallel child and adult activities. It also fosters collaboration in setting agendas for each class session. If the site sponsor, site coordinator, or project administrator is different from the training staff, they should participate in the initial training. The implementation training for new parent trainers and child program coordinators is comprised of at least 20 hours of class session. This training follows the concepts presented in the DTBY Community Training Manual and is also available from the DTBY program.

Professional qualifications vary across sites and may be influenced by the availability of college-educated individuals whose backgrounds are in human services. The parent trainer should have a bachelor's degree in a related field and previous experience with human development or parenting strategies or family life education. A master's degree is desirable. For populations that include a high percentage of non English speakers, trainers should be fluent in the language of the participants or they should co-train with someone fluent in the language. The child program coordinator should have training in early childhood development, as well as group experience with preschoolers. The ability to supervise teen helpers and work with a broad age range of children is recommended.

Programs that are in the process of replicating DTBY at new sites have found it helpful to work with existing DTBY programs during the training phase and in the early part of implementation. Existing programs can give tips on personnel qualifications, essential or core features of the program, nuts and bolts of the implementation process, how to circumvent obstacles, how to adapt curricular activities without sacrificing program fidelity (e.g., Blakely, Mayer, Gottschalk, Schmitt, Davidson, Roitman, & Emshoff, 1987), and so forth. The DTBY program maintains a list of these programs and can provide this connection to other programs at no cost.

Teen Teachers

Teens are recruited from the local community to act as Teen Angels or assistant teachers and mentors for the younger children. The number of teens recruited will depend on the number of children in the participating families. The teacher-to-student ratio should not exceed 1:5. If 25 children were enrolled, this ratio would be met with one child program coordinator and four Teen Angels.

The teens can be recruited through local agencies and schools. They should complete an application that describes how their previous experience qualifies them to be teen teachers, and it should also include the reasons they would like the job. After the program director and child program coordinator review applications, the teens are interviewed. Both of these steps focus on the motivation and the reliability of applicants. Some sites may require screening teens for any record of delinquency, sexual assault, and so forth. If teens are not screened, the program logistics must allow constant supervision by the child program coordinator. Teens should sign a contract stipulating that they will work for the complete workshop series. Because they are assigned as constant companions to individual children, the children depend on that continuity.

The Teen Angels should receive a minimum of six hours of training before they start. This training is a combination of the DTBY strategies and activities (covered in the peer and age-graded curricula described in Chapter 3), child protection strategies, and classroom management techniques. Team meetings with teens before each session continue the training process. Class plans are mutually decided upon and the activities are reviewed before each session.

Individual sites vary in the amount of responsibility that is given to the Teen Angels. In some cases, teens actually lead group and small group activities. In other instances, the teens' role is limited to helping their constant companions. All staff, including teens, should be involved in the weekly setup and cleanup of the program.

PARENT–CHILD ACTIVITIES

Parent-child (joint) activities should occur before the families divide into separate age groups for workshops. These joint activities are central to the program and need to be emphasized. In the pilot year of the original demonstration project, these activities were scheduled at the end of each workshop session, but some families would leave before or during the activity. Complete participation occurs more often when this activity is early in the session; families get to practice their new skills together under the tutelage of the staff and, pragmatically, the joint activities count toward the incentive.

Parent–child activities can be selected from a variety of sources (see Chapter 3). However they should be congruent with the theme for the session. Program staff will want to consider whether physical activities, art, projects, or a mixture of these approaches are most effective in a given group.

A sample parent–child activity for self-esteem is the song "Beautiful arms" in which parents and children act out the motions described in the song. Another activity values the family: Families make an origami house, tepee, or hogan that has pictures of the family members inside. Parents also make a flower name tag that has the child's picture inside; the petals are filled with words that the parent(s) see as positive attributes of the child.

In the area of self-responsibility, pounding playdough for anger management involves all of the family. They can also have fun creating "sculptures" out of the clay. In another session, a family version of the Feelings Cube described in Chapter 2 can create awareness of each other's feelings. Even activities like Duck-

Duck-Goose and a "literary tea," where children prepare cookies and select books for their parents to read to them, cover many of DTBY's educational objectives.

PARENT CLASSES

The parent curriculum is drawn primarily from the DTBY Parent Training Manual. The manuals include proven methods to reach the core program objectives. Unlike many curricula, however, the staff is encouraged to include creative, culture-specific activities, examples, and reinforcers that would still meet the same objectives.

Key curricular objectives are derived from the social–cognitive model described in Chapter 2. Activities also incorporate some basic child development to teach realistic expectations and how to adapt child-rearing practices in age-appropriate ways. Each class is designed to minimize lectures and to maximize activities where parents internalize the concepts and where they have input through discussion and small group exercises. Each class should include activities for different learning styles.

The sample activities described here do not constitute the entire curriculum but are representative applications of the underlying theory. The classes are described as evening programs. Daytime classes that serve lunch have also been successful. The drawback of the daytime classes, in our experience, has been that fewer fathers attend and teen educators are usually in school.

The following is an example of a typical agenda in the self-efficacy/self-esteem component:

- An introductory activity called "The M&M game" has the parents identify several of their strengths or positive characteristics. To "earn" M&Ms, they mingle and exchange positive characteristics. This warm-up activity helps the group to feel comfortable with each other and is congruent with the educational goals of the evening.
- Next is a concrete model of self-concept using the metaphor of a balloon. The rest of the sessions on self-concept, which might discuss the abstract idea of self-appraisals, build on this model. When a concrete method of defining key terms and concepts is used, parents better understand how to create structures that enhance self-esteem and self-efficacy in children and how the concepts fit together.
- Then participants are actively involved in a role-play that portrays a normal day in the life of a preschooler. This role-play illustrates the effects on a young child of everyday comments made by family and preschool staff. Usually, families are startled by the way in which many "normal" comments and actions can hurt children. Family members then make their own

"self-concept sign" and decorate it with their strengths. They are also instructed to tear off pieces when events happen during the class that degrade their feelings about themselves. They are encouraged to continue to decorate or enlarge their signs as they think of more positive characteristics or strengths.

- The first class always ends with an activity called Success Sharing. This activity is used as the first "reentry" activity in every subsequent class. As described in Chapter 2, success is redefined as all of the simple tasks a person completes or goals a person reaches during the week. Everyone participates in this activity each week. Although the norms of group work typically allow people to "pass" or not participate, this activity is the exception. Many family members have learned, as a life strategy, to "disappear" in a group setting. Sometimes this happens because it is also more comfortable for the facilitator to let that person "disappear." Therefore, Success Sharing is the one activity that is integrated so that the facilitator involves each person every week. The response can be as simple as "I made it here."
- An activity to end the program is to pass a koosh ball (or other soft, fuzzy ball) to let every person mention something that they learned from the class that night or some skill they will try during the week.

Each class has a rhythm or structure: Beginning with "Success Sharing," including a participatory activity, some didactic information, some discussion, a period to write or think silently, and a conclusion where participants give feedback about the class as a way to internalize a key concept.

Self-Efficacy/Self-Esteem

The primary learning objective for these sessions is to develop parental self-efficacy. The second objective is to give parents the skills to develop self-efficacy and self-esteem in their children. This component is placed first to follow the social–cognitive model. Strategies include the following:

- Parents identify personal strengths as a basis for building new skills. Parents become aware of their own beliefs about themselves and how those beliefs affect their child-rearing practices.
- Parents learn concepts related to self-esteem and self-efficacy.
- Parents learn factors that enhance children's self-appraisals.
- Parents learn factors that erode their self-concepts, as well as their children's.
- Parents experience strategies and activities to use with their children such as "Catch them being good," which involve giving meaningful and positive feedback to the child.
- Parents learn to help children develop their own "rudder," to evaluate themselves and not be overly dependent on external evaluation.

Self-Responsibility

This section of the curriculum focuses on recognizing and acknowledging feelings, developing an internal locus of control, family management styles that internalize locus of control, appropriate causal attributions, and stress management. Related to affect, role plays help parents learn skills to acknowledge feelings that are expressed by their children; these role plays identify common responses parents have to children's feelings. Regarding locus of control, parents review common "I can't" and "I have to" statements that are subtle statements of external control. Through a series of activities, they become aware of choices that they have made that actually are more consistent with "I won't" and "I choose to" statements. Thus, parents become aware of the way their choice of words might model internal locus of control for their children rather than helplessness or powerlessness.

A dramatization that helps parents to visualize control dynamics is "Strings." A volunteer, who plays the part of a parent, is given a pair of scissors. Ten to twelve other volunteers each receive a 10-foot piece of yarn and a "role." They play parts of family members, a person in a place of employment, or other stressors such as money, an unreliable vehicle, or self-talk. Each person ties one end of the yarn to the volunteer who plays the parent role. Before the activity begins, each person who has a string attached to the parent describes the role that person will play during the activity. Thus, a family member might scold, "You don't use good discipline with your child, he just runs wild." Their child might whine, "You never spend any time with me." A co-worker accuses, "I hear you're talking about me again." Then there's the car that needs to be fixed, the money that is too tight to afford both the phone and groceries, and the self that says, "You're no good."

When the activity starts, all of the participants simultaneously tug on the strings and shout their roles. The job of the parent under this stress is to prioritize which string is to be cut first, second, and so on. It is a very dramatic example of the stresses caused when we become externally controlled by many sources. It also is a good departure point for discussing internal versus external control dynamics in a person's life.

Causal attributions (e.g., child blame or self-blame) are formally introduced through a "time line" activity where parents decide when certain behaviors and abilities occur in youth. This approach is used because parents are more likely to make child-blaming attributions as children become more competent. They often underestimate the effect of situations on children's behavior (Dix & Grusec, 1985), and certain situations such as household hazards and potty accidents in early childhood and caving in to peer pressure in middle childhood are more likely at different ages. More often, though, parents learn to make accurate attributions in the course of group discussions when specific child-rearing issues are brought up and the group engages in problem solving. As part of the problem-solving process, the parent facilitator might ask questions about the child's goals for misbehavior, consistent with systematic training for effective parenting (STEP) (Dinkmeyer & McKay, 1976).

The "Tower Activity" is a dramatic role-play that illustrates variations in locus of control that are associated with general styles of behavior management. Three volunteers each build a tower of blocks under the watchful eye of a parent who use either an authoritarian (controlling), permissive ("whatever"), or author-itative (encouraging) approach to direct the tower building. The ensuing discussion revolves around how children (and adults) feel, believe, and act with each child-rearing style. Effective approaches that involve intrinsic motivation and reasoning are then reviewed.

Parents are taught how to set limits with input from their children, to give choices (freedom within limits), to establish win-win situations in problem solving, and to use techniques that enforce limits but still develop an internal locus of control (e.g., time-out, consequences). Parents are not criticized for the way they discipline their own children, even though they may spank, but the parent facilitators do describe the effects of different strategies on internalized control, behavior problems, and moral reasoning (see Webster-Stratton & Herbert, 1993). Democratic approaches are described—choices, consequences, reasoning, time out—as alternatives that are effective ways to foster self-regulation and prosocial behavior among children.

Decision-Making and Problem-Solving Skills

In this section of the curriculum, parents develop skills for giving children choices within the limits established by the family, for structuring situations so that children learn to solve their own problems, and for generating alternatives in difficult social situations. These conflict-resolution and negotiating skills also apply to the parents' lives. The parent facilitator models these skills when parents ask what to do about a particular child-rearing or personal concern. Staff resist the temptation to solve the participants' problems for them. Instead, the facilitator often returns the problem-solving responsibility to the parents.

Developmental patterns in moral reasoning are described, and strategies are used throughout the workshop series that encourage participants to expand their reasoning. Many activities incorporate discussion sessions where participants can express their views and the reasons for them. The participants' varied risk profiles result in different levels of reasoning and different life experiences that are factored into their reasoning. Discussions inevitably include one or two persons who reason at a slightly higher level than the rest of the class, which challenges the accepted wisdom of other participants. The resulting disequilibrium can lead to a broader perspective on the situation; facilitators often observe that some participants actually move to a higher level of reasoning on specific issues.

COMMUNICATION AND SOCIAL SKILL DEVELOPMENT

Many adults in the program find it difficult to establish good relationships with their own support systems, let alone teach their children effective social and communication skills. Other parents may have good social skills, but one of their children may struggle with making and keeping friends. The curriculum is designed to improve adults' personal relationships, to improve parent–child communication, and to help parents help their children with social skills.

Social cognition includes processes by which children understand themselves and others. An important aspect of this developmental process is social role-taking or perspective-taking, in which children learn to discriminate their own point of view from their companion's perspective and to coordinate different perspectives. For instance, with development, children realize that their relationship with their mother is different from their mother's relationship with a sibling, or that friends may have disagreements about an issue because of their differing beliefs, value systems, and expectations. As role-taking skills develop, children move from describing others in terms of external attributes to descriptions involving internal factors such as thoughts, feelings, intentions, and motives.

Robert Selman (1980) described a developmental sequence in role-taking that can help parents put their children's behavior into perspective. For example, parents often complain that their preschooler "does not listen." In many such cases, though, the child may not have the cognitive skills to understand the parent's viewpoint and what is being said. Also, young children's conflicts over possessions often are due to their egocentrism. These normal conflicts are described in The Toddler's Creed, attributed to Burton White, which says in part, "If I want it, it's mine. If I can take it away from you, it's mine. If I had it a little while ago, it's mine." Parent concerns can thus be alleviated if they realize that communication failures and social conflicts are due to their children's normal egocentrism.

The actual age at which children experience Selman's stages will vary:

- *Stage 0*: Egocentric, undifferentiated social perspective taking (3 to 6 years). Children cannot make clear distinctions between their own interpretation of a situation and another's point of view. They have difficulty recognizing that their own perspective may be incorrect.
- *Stage 1*. Differentiated, subjective perspective taking (5 to 9 years). Although children begin to realize that others may have different points of view, they may not fully or accurately understand these views. They may believe that these views are different from their own because other people are privy to different information.
- *Stage 2*. Self-reflective, reciprocal perspective-taking (7 to 12 years). Chil-

dren can reflect on their own thoughts and feelings from another's perspective, but they cannot hold both their own perspective and that of another person simultaneously.

- *Stage 3*. Third person or mutual perspective-taking (10 to 15 years). Adolescents can step outside their own and others' perspectives to assume the perspective of a neutral third person. Now they can simultaneously consider their own point of view and can recognize that another person can do the same. Therefore, friendships tend to become more than mutual back scratching, and conflicts can be viewed in terms of mutual differences.
- *Stage 4*. In-depth and societal perspective-taking (adolescence to adulthood). Individuals become aware that motives, thoughts, and actions can be shaped by psychological factors. Social perspective-taking is often on a more abstract level that involves a generalized societal perspective. The maturation in role-taking skills and empathy allows for more mature self-understanding, friendships, group participation, and parent/adolescent relationships.

Ironically, many adult participants in the program have not yet reached Stage 4. Thus, although the workshop activities are intended to help parents work with their children, they may actually help the parents to expand their perspective-taking abilities.

This section of the curriculum includes skill-building activities for perspective-taking such as recognizing feelings in oneself and others. One example of this is a role-taking activity where parents play the role of a child to help them relate to the child's perspective. They wear large bulky gloves, and a rather demanding "parent" expects the child to color, cut, and open a tiny box of raisins quickly and neatly.

Parents also learn how value systems guide communication patterns. In interactions with other people, communication skills usually are applied in one of two ways: to get my own way, which involves altering others' behavior, or to gain and keep healthy relationships, which establishes equal value between two parties. Although both are valid strategies depending on the circumstance, people who are just learning communication skills often unconsciously adopt the first strategy, "to get my own way." Adult family members are encouraged to use new skills to create open, equal communication that values each person's needs and perspectives.

Within this context, skills for using I-messages and reflective listening are practiced and modeled. The concept of assertive, aggressive, and passive communication styles is introduced. The implications of each style for healthy relationships are explored. Parents even learn basic "resistance skills." This is important for them in their own relationships, and it is also important for them as role models to their children.

FUTURE ORIENTATION

The ability to see oneself playing a positive role in the future has been well-documented as a resiliency factor. This is important for both children and their parents. In one of the first sessions of the family classes, parents are asked to identify a goal they have for themselves in one year and in five years. The fact that a large percentage of the adult family members struggle with this concept emphasizes its importance. They are also asked to identify a goal they have for the focal child in one year. This list of goals, without names attached, is posted in the classroom, so that facilitators can link the different skills covered in the class with individual goals.

Classroom environment surveys show that participants believe that the information and skills learned are important and have improved their child-rearing practices, as well as adult relationships. Participants also like the workshops because their experiences are normalized—other parents share the same trials and tribulations—and a social support system develops.

Although the parent curriculum is designed for families with 2- to 5-year-old children, the basic concepts are applicable to parents of all ages. The program materials, combined with the school curriculum, have been adapted for family classes and children of all ages. The DTBY program has applied these strategies to families that have children 6 to 11 years old and found that both parents and children make improvements in their communication and self-efficacy; child-rearing practices also improve.

The concepts have also been applied successfully in a family approach to juvenile diversion for youth from 10 to 18 years old. In many communities, youth who have committed their first or second offense are referred to a diversion program. These youth can be "diverted" from the court system, and the record expunged, if remedial action such as public service and educational programs for the offending youth is taken. The DTBY family concept includes another alternative. Youth must attend 20 hours of DTBY classes. A fee is charged unless the youth bring parents to each class. If parents attend, the fee is waived. In the first five years of the project, 95% of the referred youth were accompanied by parents. The importance of involving the family in such interventions is becoming more apparent. Data show that recidivism drops significantly for youth in the program compared to youth who are not in the program. Surveys of both parents and youth also show significant increases in skills that are consistent with the data reported in this monograph for preschool families.

Therefore, DTBY represents a resource that can be used in communities that want to provide a family-based empowerment program for youth of any age. The program is made even more flexible because it can be adapted to many cultural backgrounds.

DARE to be You Community Team and School Training

Research on the ecology of risk-taking behavior in youth, as well as on effective preventive approaches, clearly demonstrates the importance of involving multiple microsystems that surround youth and families. Establishing links among the different microsystems and building positive links between families and the settings in which they are embedded is vitally important to a comprehensive prevention program.

COMMUNITY TRAINING TO SUPPORT THE DARE TO BE YOU FAMILY/PRESCHOOL PROGRAM

The DTBY program has addressed this ecological issue through a team training strategy. If the community training supports a particular target audience, as it would in the program for families with 2- to 5-year-old youth, it is important to invite representatives from key agencies in the community that serve those families. Ideally 15 to 40 community members participate together in a 15-hour interactive training program held in their community. The recommended composition of community team training includes representatives from a minimum of six agencies or organizations in the community. In addition to the educational goals of community training, the experience is designed to create a supportive network among the agencies and with the families. Community team members learn about the DTBY program's research base and its educational objectives for the families. Therefore, it contributes to a broad-based referral network as team members learn about DTBY and each other's efforts and become committed to these principles of effective prevention. The community training also enhances a sense of support among participants and expands their capacities to help.

Many different agencies have either sponsored or participated in community training that is designed to support the program for families with 2- to 5-year-old youth. These agencies include social services, mental health, education, family centers, urban leagues, Head Start, preschools, substance abuse treatment or prevention centers, health department personnel, home visitor programs, and youth shelter personnel.

Community Team Training as Capacity Building for Working with Youth

The DTBY community training was originally developed as a resource to build capacity for youth workers. The community, or sponsoring agencies, identifies the target populations and organizes the training around the specific needs of that community. An important consideration in any context is that representatives from multiple agencies participate. The actual makeup of the trained team will vary with the needs identified in a given community. It has included representatives from law enforcement; kindergarten, elementary, middle, and high school teachers and counselors; community youth-group leaders (4-H, Scouts, Campfire Girls); church youth-group leaders; staff for after-school programs; mental health, social services, and health department personnel; YMCA and YWCA; recreation departments; camp personnel; and health care providers.

Educational Objectives of Community Team Training

Three approaches are included in the community team-training format. Participants learn strategies to enhance the ability of youth to attain the educational goals of the project. Participants also discuss ways to create positive environments in working with youth that enhance their development. Finally, participants experience sample activities from the preschool, school-age, adolescent, and parent curriculum. The specific activities selected depend on the target age group of the community team.

The training follows the same outline for social–cognitive development as described in Chapter 2 and illustrated for youth and families in Chapters 3 and 4. Thus, participants learn about developing self-efficacy and self-esteem, responsibility, decision making and problem solving, and communication/social skills. Participants are trained to use the activities in the curriculum materials outlined in Chapters 3 and 4. However, the curriculum manuals do not contain the theoretical and scientific grounding of each activity nor the strategies and environmental factors that are covered in the implementation training.

DARE TO BE YOU STRATEGIES

Development of efficacy is a key theoretical concept for the entire program. Therefore, an important strategy is to strengthen the efficacy of the participants in the community team training. The training models the process to be used with clients. Team members might be taught by example ways to encourage participation when youth are learning a new skill. A volunteer is asked to come to the front of the class and "draw a rose" on a flipchart, choosing from a selection of colored markers. The usual scenario is that no one volunteers immediately; the facilitator simply waits, and someone eventually does volunteer. The volunteer is thanked and encouraged to proceed. Then, the focus turns to all of the participants who did not volunteer. The facilitator asks the "audience" to think of the reasons that they did not volunteer. The usual answers include "I can't draw," "I was afraid I wouldn't make it look like you wanted it to look," "My mother (teacher, sibling) told me I couldn't draw," or "I'm not an artist." The audience is challenged to look at the origin and the validity of those beliefs. They are also asked to consider the standard against which they are evaluating themselves.

When the volunteer finishes her "rose," the facilitator makes a valid, positive comment. The volunteer is asked why she volunteered. The usual reply has to do with positive art experiences or confidence in drawing ability. The point is that one result of our very product-oriented society can be to neglect the importance of the process side of learning. Although the finished product is important, the learning process should also be valued.

In the case of the rose, people's beliefs are based on an evaluation of a product—their picture. Either an early experience made them believe that their "product" was not good enough, or they thought they had to "produce" something that met a certain standard. When applied to all situations, these beliefs can really inhibit efficacy development, motivation, and creativity. However, each person in the room may have been able to create a picture of a rose that communicated their feelings or experiences with that flower, which is the process component of the activity. Participants are challenged to think of specific cases where the process can be valued in their particular circumstances of working with youth. A classic example is grading in school systems. In most classes, grades are given for a certain level of mastery—the level of knowledge is a product. Some children may come into the class already knowing 90% of the material. They learn 5% more and get an A for their 95%. Other children may come into the class knowing only 40% of the material; they learn 35% and achieve a 75% level. They have actually learned seven times what was learned by the A student but receive a C.

This type of grading system is very effective at measuring existing competencies (product) but does not value the advancement (process).

Another example of the product/process dilemma is the pressure that parents of preschool youth often feel to "evaluate" a child's picture. "What a pretty ... uh, uh, um ..." as the parent struggles to correctly identify the drawing's content. This type of evaluation emphasizes the "product." However, parents can also comment on how much the child enjoyed coloring, choosing colors, or making big motions—the process.

A concrete model is also used to introduce some of the concepts in the area of self-responsibility. Marionettes are likened to youth as they mature. There is the "star puppet" stage where children are fairly compliant and parents or teachers control the strings (in early and late childhood). Even so, children at this age may also have "berserk strings" that might be pulled by siblings and others. Starting in early adolescence, youth may enter the "Pinocchio stage" where they want to be "real people," not puppets, and they want to take their strings back from parents and other caregivers. This is described as a risky stage if the youth do not realize that they have strings or have not developed any skills to pull those strings. The strings are just "laying around" for whomever might decide to pick them up, usually "honest Johns" who do not have the adolescent's best interests in mind.

An example activity related to self-responsibility is to have team members look at the subtle messages given to youth by adults about internal versus the external locus of control. Adults often say, "I have to ..." (go to work, pay the bills, clean the house). This subtly suggests an external attribution for behavior. These comments send the message that the adult is externally controlled in some unidentified way and that it is appropriate for adults to be externally controlled. Participants are taught to look at their "I have to" statements, devise seven alternatives for a given situation, and examine the alternatives' consequences. After doing this, participants often realize that the statements actually are choices that a person has made for very good reasons; they are internally controlled. This can change people's perception of their locus of control and make them more aware of the message such statements can send. Youth may learn only the message conveyed by language, so adults in their lives are challenged to examine their real "strings" and to make the message and the actual experience more congruent.

A sample strategy related to problem solving and decision making is to avoid the traps of "judging" and "fixing." Role-play activities show traps that people can fall into when they try to fix problems for youth. Participants are encouraged to use problem-solving and conflict-resolution strategies that encourage youth to participate in problem solving. This means that students generate their own choices, and adults do not give them the ideas.

Regarding communication strategies, participants need to be aware of comments or responses that adults use to imply that children cannot trust their own feelings or that their feelings are not valid or important. Examples of such comments include, "You don't really feel that way," "Life is just like that," or "You must have done something first to cause the problem." Participants learn more appropriate strategies that acknowledge the child's feelings without blaming them or being too quick to offer solutions (see Faber & Mazlish, 1980).

Ideas for Creating a Positive Environment

The overall environment is vitally important to successful prevention or educational programs for youth. Participants in the community training learn how to structure positive yet controlled learning situations. Some of the ideas are simple "think ahead" clues to make activities work. Even simple activities can have pitfalls, such as identifying a positive characteristic in another person and making an "award" for it. If a group of 10 year olds is assigned to make awards for other children in the class and any person may give anyone else an award, what might happen? The most popular children will probably receive the lion's share of the awards. Some rejected children who already have low self-esteem may get no awards. This creates a situation where the children who could really benefit from this activity really end up wounded by it. An alternative that is both fair and effective is to let students work in pairs or small groups to give each other the awards.

This example illustrates the importance of setting norms in a group of youth in a way that creates a sense of safety and motivation. To be congruent with the DTBY model, participants learn to set norms based on input from the class. A list of proposed ideas is voted on by the class (using thumbs up or down). Participants can ask for clarification of proposals before voting. One person voting against a norm can remove it from consideration, unless an amendment is suggested. Of course, the group leader may have some nonnegotiable norms that have to be added at the end (see Webster-Stratton & Herbert, 1993). This usually does not happen if the input and voting procedures are implemented effectively.

This standard norm-setting procedure should not end with voting on group rules. To be effective, the group should also decide what the consequences will be for violating the agreed–upon norms. As before, this is involves brainstorming and reaching consensus. In the last step, the group decides how to use good communication skills to tell "offenders" that they have committed infractions. Although this is standard practice in many settings, youth workers often have not been trained to use basic, positive management strategies. It is a key element in establishing a positive learning environment because it promotes self-responsibility and an internalized locus of control.

In summary, the community training adheres to the same social–cognitive theory that was described in previous chapters. Educational exercises are primarily experiential, supplemented by discussion with some didactic information. An essential feature is that valuing others and problem-solving and communication skills are modeled through all training modules.

SCHOOL TRAINING

The school is a powerful microsystem for youth and families from preschool into adulthood. In keeping with ecological systems theory, a comprehensive prevention program needs to have a component that involves schools. The DTBY program addresses the school's role with a component that is designed to develop teacher efficacy and to enhance the school's educational and interpersonal environment. This curriculum also includes activities for teachers to use with youth. As before, the activities and intervention process are guided by social–cognitive theory (see Chapters 1 and 2).

School Component to Support the DARE to be You Family Program

Head Start staff, preschool teachers, and day-care providers make up the school microsystem for 2- to 5-year-old children and their families. Their qualifications, training, and experience often are extremely varied. Yet research demonstrates that these early caregivers exert a powerful influence on children; the quality of early child-care settings is strongly related to young children's emotional and cognitive development (NICHD, 1999; Peisner-Feinberg & Burchinal, 1997). Therefore, in the DTBY program for families with preschoolers, a special effort was made to involve the teachers of the children in the program. Because of the very diverse community settings, sponsoring organizations, and approaches at the sites in which the program was originally tested, the mechanisms to involve the "school" setting varied widely.

Two of the original four sites were actually sponsored by a preschool agency: an urban multi-service child-care center in Colorado Springs and the Native American site. At each of these sites, the sponsoring agency included DTBY staff training as part of their regular professional development activities. In these two sites, staff training was repeated or expanded over the five years of the program. Teachers in these settings had a very strong conceptual understanding of the DTBY program theory and practice. Many of the teachers incorporated the strategies and activities into their own classrooms. These agencies also provided the workshop space for the program.

Overall, the staff was very supportive in giving access to the facilities, recruiting families, and providing many important elements of the program such as connections to other community agencies. Both program directors had been involved in the initial grant proposal and were invested in the project concept and success of the program. At the urban site, two of the preschool staff also served as children's program coordinators over the course of the pilot project. As such, there was a very strong link between the family and the school microsystems.

A different approach was adopted at the rural San Luis Valley site. Here, the Cooperative Extension Service was the primary site sponsor after the pilot year of the demonstration project. This particular office had strong connections with many community agencies, including the local Head Start and other preschool programs. Day-care and Head Start programs were involved as referral agencies, and training was provided for any day-care and Head Start teachers who wanted to attend. Although there was not as much articulation between the families and preschools at this site, compared to the two sites described earlier, individual DTBY families' teachers and child care providers were targeted. The fourth community exhibited an even looser connection between families in the program and the preschool settings because day-care and preschool teachers were involved only through the community training. However, several of the preschool and Head Start staff at this site also had children in the DTBY program, and so they participated in the training as parents.

Despite these differences in family-school partnerships and teacher training, few site differences emerged in program impact. This might suggest that family-school collaboration can be structured in a variety of ways. It may also indicate that the school piece is not as influential as the family program in altering the tested constructs, at least in preschool. However, we did not assess school readiness directly nor attitudes toward learning environments, which might have been more favorable at the Colorado Springs and Native American sites. Also, we believe that stronger family-school collaboration early in development empowers parents to be more proactive with teachers once their children enter elementary school, a hypothesis that remains to be tested.

The training format also varied by community. The common thread was that teachers and care providers for the 2- to 5-year-old youth received at least 15 hours of training. This training was distributed across two consecutive days of workshops in some cases, whereas teachers at other sites participated in weekly in-service training that lasted 2 to 4 hours each. The content of the training followed the same conceptual outline described for the community training with adaptations for specific preschool and day-care environments. For example, to learn how to establish group norms, teachers would use puppets to act out scenarios that depicted appropriate and inappropriate behaviors and then would ask the preschoolers to vote with thumbs up or thumbs down. This is a more concrete method than the approach for older children, which entails brainstorming and discussion to consensus. Teachers were encouraged to use many of the activities from the DTBY preschool curriculum.

School Components for Elementary, Middle, and High School Programs

Teacher efficacy is a primary objective of the training at every age level. Research on the teacher-training component showed that teachers who participated in the training program and who actually used the curriculum demonstrated significant gains in teacher efficacy and satisfaction with their role (Fritz et al., 1995). They also showed decreases in indicators for burnout. These psychosocial characteristics of teachers have a significant bearing on the quality of the school environment.

Teacher training parallels the community training. They participate in at least 15 hours of class, which guides them in implementing strategies in the classroom and modifying the broader school environment. Teachers may use the curriculum designed for grades K–12, or they may simply incorporate the strategies into their existing classrooms. Teacher feedback indicates that the flexibility of the DTBY curriculum gives them the necessary latitude to implement activities in creative ways, as well as to develop their own approaches that suit their teaching styles.

The Impact of DARE to be You

A recent review of programs for parents noted that few family-based intervention programs had been systematically evaluated (Cowan et al., 1998). Previous evaluations had not used samples that were large enough to detect program effects, few included no-treatment or alternative treatment control groups, much less random assignment to groups, and few used multiple measures and methods to reduce bias. Cowan et al. (1998) also decried the lack of long-term follow-ups that would reveal whether program effects were ephemeral. These authors noted that interventions may create disequilibrium in the family system at first, but in the long run, effective programs result in "reorganization at a new structural level" (p. 56). Thus, "sleeper effects" may be fairly common. As parents wrestle with new ideas, try out new approaches, and figure out what works and what doesn't, positive outcomes may emerge or be strengthened with the passage of time.

Our evaluation of DTBY was mindful of these flaws in prior studies of family-based programs. We recruited a large number of families so that we had adequate power to detect even small program effects. Families were assigned at random to the intervention and control groups and then were followed for as long as three years. And sleeper effects were found in some areas, particularly in parents' causal attributions. Finally, we used multiple measures for several of the core constructs, particularly parent self-appraisals and child-rearing practices. Following sound evaluation practice (Rossi & Freeman, 1989), we also described how DTBY was implemented, so that others could replicate the program and so that we could document how the program was adapted for diverse groups.

The sections that follow are organized around key questions that guided the program's evaluation. First, we describe the participants with particular attention to risk status, sample size, and attrition. Next we describe how the program was implemented and how both DTBY staff and local community agencies perceived the program. The third section describes how program impact was measured and what we found. The final section describes our search for individual differences in program impact, in which we examine age and risk profiles. Such individual differences can be important because different "types" of people may benefit from different intervention approaches.

WHO PARTICIPATED IN THE PROGRAM EVALUATION?

A total of 496 intervention and 301 control parents began the initial high-risk demonstration project. Five cohorts were recruited, and between 84 and 182 parents took part in each yearly wave. We did not include data from the initial pilot year because the groups were not assigned at random at one site, the curriculum was not implemented as designed at one site, and neither the curriculum nor the evaluative tools were finalized. In subsequent years, families who met the risk profile (see later) and who had children between 2 and 5 years of age were assigned at random to the DTBY program or the control group.

How Were Families Recruited into the Program?

Families were referred to DTBY by community agencies. These included county departments of health, mental health, and social services; housing agencies; the court system; family physicians; the Urban League; and school, Head Start, and day-care programs. After the first year, recommendations from families who participated in the program led to many self-referrals. Of those recruited, fewer than 5% refused their group assignment or dropped out before completing the DTBY program.

What Risk Factors Did the Families Have?

Family risk was defined by the criteria listed in Table 4.1, all of which have been linked to later adolescent substance use (Hawkins et al., 1992). A composite risk index combining these variables showed that the average parent had three risk factors at entry into the program; 73% had one to four major risk factors present, and 22% had five or more.

A majority of the families was at risk because of economic disadvantage (59%) or family history of substance abuse (42% to 55% of the parents reported that relatives had a drinking problem), yet few were so troubled that they should have been referred to therapy. The goal was to recruit some families with no risk factors (7.2% had none). This helps to include diverse role models in each group and to avoid stigmatizing participants. Another goal was to select families with acute rather than severe, chronic difficulties that might require therapy. Thus, the program staff was successful in recruiting families from the target population that met the desired risk profile.

A majority of the families were from low-income or blue-collar backgrounds. The median annual family income was $14,500, and 45% received some form of welfare. The typical wage earner was an unskilled laborer or service worker. Parent educational attainment varied between 7 and 22 years ($M = 12.7$); 26.4% were high school dropouts. This was an ethnically diverse sample: 22% Hispanic, 29% Native American, 2% African-American, and 45% Anglo. Most of the participants were either married (53.7%) or cohabiting (10.7%); the rest were single (15%), separated (7%), or divorced (12.6%). The mothers averaged 29.7 years of age, and the fathers 31.5 years of age. The women had their first children at an average age of 22.2 years (30% as teenagers), and their youngest child was 3.15 years of age. Less than 3% of the families had children placed in foster care in the previous year. Finally, less than one in five participants had sought individual or family therapy in the previous six months, but there were systematic variations in such help seeking. Anglo caregivers were more likely to access such community resources, even when controlling for income, self-efficacy, and social supports.

How Did the Sites Differ?

The DTBY program was implemented in four sites that differed markedly in their social ecology. These four sites will be referred to as the Native American (Ute Mountain Ute) site, the San Luis Valley site, the Montezuma County site, and the Colorado Springs site. These differences were important to test the replicability of the intervention program across cultures and degrees of community risk. The **Native American Site** was in the Four Corners area and was more than 95% Native American. This was considered an at-risk community because of the high rate of teen parents and substance abuse problems among youth. At the inception of the program, there were high rates of unemployment and school dropout. The average life expectancy was 37.8 years. Both the Native American site and the San Luis Valley site are isolated rural areas where there are few people scattered over large areas.

The **San Luis Valley site** included 43% Hispanic families, many of whom traced their ancestry to the conquistadors. Of the Hispanic parents in our sample, 67% live in this area. An economically depressed region, it has a high unemployment rate, the lowest per capita income in Colorado, and a high rate of farm foreclosures. At the time the project started, nearly 10% of pregnant women received inadequate prenatal care; rates of teen pregnancy, child abuse, and DUI filings were in the top decile for Colorado; and only 35% of Hispanic adults in the San Luis Valley were high school graduates, compared to 78.6% of adults in the state.

The **Montezuma County site** is a semirural area in the southwestern high desert. Like the San Luis Valley site, this site has high rates of unemployment and poverty, and higher than average rates of substance abuse and child abuse. Few services are available for low-income families: only one licensed infant day care; no prenatal parenting classes; few mental health or addictions programs, especially for parents; and no follow-up support programs for teen parents. The population in this area is predominately Anglo, Hispanic, and Native American.

In contrast, the **Colorado Springs (Urban) site**, with a population of 281,000, provides much greater access to support services for parents. However, a highly transient populace and polarization along SES lines have eroded the sense of community. This city has among the highest rates of child abuse and teen pregnancy in the state.

There are also other indicators of diversity across sites. Families at the County site were the most advantaged because more parents were married, fewer received welfare payments, they made more money per year, and they were older. In contrast, the Native American site may have been the most at risk because of low annual incomes, lower educational attainment, and the reported high rates of alcoholism, although this risk is somewhat offset by their strong support networks. The sites did differ on the cumulative risk score; the Colorado Springs and Native American sites had significantly higher scores than the other two sites. Such family risk and sample diversity provide a strong test of how well the prevention program works with families of diverse needs and backgrounds.

How Were Families Followed over Time?

Caregivers (usually parents) and other family members completed a set of baseline measures before they were assigned to groups. Those in the intervention group completed post-test measures when the workshops were completed, typically three months after baseline. The post-test was not administered to control families to reduce costs—it is difficult for testers to track down families one at a time in these rural areas—and because we did not expect much change in the controls after only three months. Caregivers in both groups then completed follow-up measures at one-year intervals after the baseline.

The retention rate for attendance in the first series of classes met our goal of 95%. Few caregivers (5%) dropped out of the project between baseline and the completion of the workshops. The retention rate was 75% at the one-year follow-up and 71% at the two-year follow-up. These retention rates, combined with the large sample size, provide a high level of statistical power (.90) to detect fairly small intervention effects (ES = .25).

Attrition poses a problem if it is selective because those who remain in the study may differ in important ways from those who do not complete follow-up measures. To test for selective attrition, we divided all participants into those who had completed the second follow-up questionnaires versus those who had dropped out of the study. These two groups were compared on a number of baseline demographic variables (e.g., age, education, income), as well as on various measures of parenting and child development. The groups were similar on all but three variables when they entered the program, indicating that selective attrition was not an issue. It *is* interesting that in the original trial as well as in a later replication, age was one of the few initial variables that related to attrition: younger mothers were more likely to drop out.

HOW WAS DARE TO BE YOU IMPLEMENTED?

Systematic knowledge of the way a program is implemented is essential to understanding program outcomes, as well as to guiding replication efforts (King, Morris, & Fitz-Gibbon, 1987). Program impact may vary with the "dosage" participants receive. If a program is not implemented with fidelity, it is also less likely to have the intended impact. Finally, information about implementation guides replications and helps to distinguish core program features that must be replicated faithfully from those that can be adapted to local circumstances (Price, Cowen, Lorion, & Ramos-McKay, 1989). The issue of fidelity is particularly salient when providing intervention services to diverse families because Native American, Hispanic, and Anglo belief systems and languages are likely to influence receptivity of the families to certain materials and messages.

We documented program implementation in a variety of ways. Throughout each workshop series, the project director and site staff documented attendance, which activities from the curriculum were given, and impressions of the way the sessions went. This was done with weekly workshop logistic worksheets. In a later replication, we used implementation logbooks to collect more systematic data on the way the curriculum was implemented and modified. Both of these methods provided a rich source of information about which activities tended to be emphasized at each site, how the time was distributed, the degree to which participants were engaged or invested in the program, and how curriculum activities were adapted for different cultures. Curiously, though, there were no consistent relations between the measures of implementation and the amount of benefit received from the program. The records also documented the dosage that each participant received. The actual number of hours of attendance was tracked for all adult participants through sign-in sheets. Adult participants were not considered to have completed the program until they had attended at least 20 hours of the workshops and parent-child activities. This indicates that the amount of exposure to the program may actually have a higher impact that which specific activities were covered.

At the posttest, the participants completed the Classroom Environment Scale, which assessed the interpersonal dynamics and task orientation of their group. They also rated their satisfaction with the program and completed open-ended questions on aspects of the program that they liked best or would change. Exit interviews were conducted with program staff that focused on the screening process, aspects of the curriculum that were more or less successful, and impressions of what made DTBY successful. The staff also completed concept maps that capture the essential features of the DTBY program. Finally, we surveyed community agencies for their impressions of the program.

How Did Participants Perceive the Program?

When asked about their global perceptions of the program, participants were uniformly enthusiastic about the workshops. When asked how much they liked the workshops and learned from them, the average ratings were 3.80 where 4 is the highest possible score. The open-ended comments were coded for major themes, and the results are reported in Table 6.1. There is convergence between parents' perceptions of what was most helpful and the changes that were found on the questionnaires. Many of those involved in the workshops thought that they had learned new parenting techniques, as indeed was the case, and that they were more self-confident, which converges with survey results on self-appraisals. Parents in the intervention group also became more satisfied with their social networks as a result of DTBY. This squares with participants' comments about normalizing parenting problems and building support systems. Most participants would not change anything in the workshops. The most common improvement suggested was to have an even more intensive or extended program. The participants who commented on accessibility most often had to drive long distances to attend, reflecting the difficulty of providing services to rural families. Some thought that the sessions were scheduled at an inconvenient time.

Participants also rated the workshops favorably on the Classroom Environment Scale (CES; Moos & Trickett, 1987). The CES assessed the group dynamics of the workshops, namely, how much the group stayed focused on educational tasks and how much effort went into making it a cohesive, supportive group. The CES has acceptable internal consistencies and test–retest correlations, and the scores on it correlate with direct observations of classroom activities and teacher behavior (Moos & Trickett, 1987).

The Task Orientation (CES) scores were very favorable; the average score ($M = 9.88$) was 79% of the maximum possible. Responses were even more positive on the Relationship scale ($M = 12.89$), which was 93% of the maximum.

Table 6.1. Participant Perceptions
of the DARE to Be You Classes

Theme	%[a]
"The best part of the workshop was …"	
Everything	3.3
Learning new parenting techniques	37.0
Normalizing parenting problems	30.8
Building support systems	34.6
Self-awareness; self-confidence	17.6
Better understanding of my child	11.0
Specific educational activities	15.8
Program provisions (child care; food; incentives)	2.6
"The part of the workshop I would change is …"	
Nothing	45.4
Offer more workshops; more intensive	17.5
Less repetitive; more goal-directed	3.5
More hands-on (active) practice; homework	3.1
Problems with group dynamics	2.6
More accessible (scheduling; proximity)	5.7
Recruit more (diverse) participants	1.7
More time for (personal) discussion	3.1
More information on specific topics	3.5
Stress reduction/anger control techniques	0.4

[a]Percentages total more than 100% because multiple responses could
be coded.

Negative correlations between the Relationship score and global perceptions of
the workshops ($r = -.34$) indicate that when participants believed that the groups
were less supportive, they were less likely to perceive the workshops as beneficial.
Some site differences on the CES were observed at the posttest but these washed
out at the Year 1 follow-up. To foreshadow findings presented later, no site differences in program impact were observed either.

How Did the DTBY Staff View the Program?

Exit interviews were conducted with the staff from all four sites to assess
their perceptions of the program. Three parent program leaders, two children's
program leaders, and one site-level program administrator were interviewed.
When asked what had attracted them originally to seek a position with DTBY, the
staff noted DTBY's focus on individual strengths and on prevention. When asked
to compare DTBY's approach with that used by other human service agencies, the
staff mentioned DTBY's greater reliance on a preventive approach, the use of
activities and hands-on experiences as opposed to lectures, clear role modeling by

the staff, and more focus on proactive problem solving compared to focusing on problems. They also stressed DTBY's emphasis on creating a supportive milieu through accepting and validating differences and feelings, and on the empathy for parents exhibited by all of the staff.

The typical staff member's educational background included at least a bachelor's degree in the behavioral or social sciences. Half of the staff had trained directly for human service agency work, and the other half came to the field via work experiences and other educational backgrounds. All staff members interviewed stressed personal family experiences that helped them to empathize with the issues and concerns of the families they served; this emotional connection was emphasized as much as their formal educational backgrounds, and may explain participants' and community members' high regard for the staff. Involvement with the DTBY program enhanced their confidence, leadership, teaching skills, and competence as parents.

The staff members were asked to consider what they had learned about families and their ability to change. The most prevalent theme was the power of focusing on individual family strengths. When the staff helps parents to recognize and work on areas of strength and support each family's own goals, the family invests the effort needed, and positive change occurs. This theme of building strengths or resilience was pervasive in staff comments about being respectful of clients and believing in the ability of individuals and families to make desired changes, if given support.

This optimistic orientation toward resilience may explain the staff's discomfort with a question about how to distinguish between screening judgments ("Which applicants are at such high risk that they need therapy rather than prevention?") and being judgmental, or stereotyping families on the basis of their high risk. Their struggles to address the question lent support to their deeply held values of focusing on family strengths, that every family faces problems and must learn to handle them, and that a positive, supportive approach is what is needed from program leaders. Few of the staff could articulate attributes that they thought would prevent families from benefiting from DTBY. Instead, the staff quickly shifted the focus to factors that help families to change. Their comments so clearly mirrored DTBY's expressed values and concepts that it was evident the staff would be likely to model them in interactions with family participants.

How Was the Program Perceived by Community Agencies?

Family service agencies in each targeted community were surveyed with regard to the impact of DTBY on the broader community; 33 of 43 agencies returned the forms. We scored agencies' knowledge of DTBY on a four-point scale; the average was 2.96, indicating that most agencies were well-informed as to the program's goals and concepts. A large majority of the agencies (73%) gave a clear description of the program or had been involved with it directly at some level.

Agency personnel said that the main strengths of the DTBY program were the curriculum (98%) and the staff (29%). Structural aspects, including child care, incentive pay, and follow-up sessions, were mentioned by 68% of the respondents, and 10% mentioned its cultural sensitivity. Agency personnel most often indicated that families gained better parenting skills, improved their family functioning, developed a stronger support system, and enhanced parental self-esteem. In terms of impact on the broader community, 87% of the agencies commented on the cooperative networking of agencies fostered by DTBY or, more commonly, that by strengthening families, DTBY played a significant role in reducing or preventing family problems. No agency reported any perceived problems or negative effects of the program, either for families or for community efforts. Thus, both inside and outside observers of DTBY reached consensus on the key program elements that were effective.

What Key DTBY Concepts Should Be Transmitted for Program Replication?

Model programs need to be able to communicate the essence of their intervention to others, so that replications can have the intended impact, ideally using the same mechanisms of change. Concept mapping provides one way to document the essence of a program. Such information is crucial in preserving the fidelity of a program because new programs should adhere to the original program's theory of change and at the same time adapt or "reinvent" program procedures for local populations (Bauman, Stein, & Ireys, 1991; Blakely et al., 1987). The DTBY impact model was discussed in the first two chapters of this monograph. The concept maps that the DTBY staff devised are a formal way to describe these mechanisms and others that are essential to the program's success.

The procedures for doing concept mapping are described by Trochim and his colleagues (Shern, Trochim, & LaComb, 1995; Trochim, 1989). First, the staff from several sites brainstormed phrases that describe specific activities, functions, or components of the DTBY program. Up to 100 descriptors were generated. Next, the staff individually sorted these descriptors into clusters that made sense to them and rated the importance of each item to DTBY. Multidimensional scaling and cluster analysis were used to combine the individual sorts into a two-dimensional map; descriptors that were often placed in the same pile by the staff were adjacent to each other in this map. The final step entailed the staff reaching consensus on titles for the clusters on this map.

The final concept map is described in the following bulleted list. Clusters that are adjacent to each other in the circular map are perceived as sharing more commonalities than clusters on opposite sides of the map. A full description along with a visual representation is being prepared for publication and will be available from the authors.

- *Value the parent role.* These items focus on normalizing parenting issues, providing good role models, supporting the parent role, and fostering improved parenting.
- *Teach parents life skills.* Descriptors in this cluster concern specific child-rearing skills and goals, such as unconditional positive regard, being an advocate for the child, making sure that parents following through with promises and actions, and having empathy for children and the way they think. Also included are life skills such as teaching parents to believe in themselves and to recognize their own successes.
- *Nurture efficacy beliefs.* Items include teaching self-responsibility rather than blaming, fostering self-worth, building resiliency and flexibility, and enhancing self-esteem as well as social skills. These items pertain to both parents and children and are congruent with Bandura's (1986) theory.
- *Develop parent–child relationships.* These descriptors focused on specific outcomes such as good communication skills, assertiveness, self-awareness, recognizing feelings, mutual respect, decision-making and problem-solving skills, and coping skills that result in an internal locus of control. All of these outcomes were seen as serving to improve family and peer relationships.
- *Enhance family strengths and pride.* Here, the staff emphasized getting the whole family involved, building healthy families, encouraging families to have fun together, teaching acceptance of each other, and building a sense of pride. That is, a family systems approach is seen as essential.
- *Supportive group environment.* This cluster focused on the nuts and bolts of how the DTBY program is implemented. Examples include using the Teen Angels and DTBY staff to model effective communication and problem-solving techniques, helping the group to take charge, and creating a safe atmosphere in which to practice new skills. The staff was cautioned against imposing their own expectations and values but instead need to be nonjudgmental and to be inclusive of family cultures.
- *Community connection and support.* Descriptors included both the outreach aspect of DTBY—to create linkages among families, schools, and community support systems—as well as fostering support networks in the family classes.

Replication sites in Utah and California generated similar concept maps with one exception: awareness of culture and diversity emerged as a distinct cluster at these sites. The similarity in the concept maps across sites, as well as the congruence between the maps and the impact theory described in Chapters 1 and 2, indicates that the DTBY staffs are well versed in the presumptions and practices of the program.

Concept maps have utility beyond capturing the essence of a program's theory and practice. For example, they can be used to guide training so that different sessions are devoted to each cluster. Concept maps can also guide program planning. Program directors can use them to assess aspects of the program that need to be strengthened with additional resources such as funding or personnel, or to discern where existing community services are duplicated and which unique niche is filled by the program (see Trochim, 1989).

DID DARE TO BE YOU HAVE AN IMPACT ON FAMILIES?

Program impact was assessed with a battery of parent-report measures. Parents selected one child (called the target or focus child) between 2 and 5 years of age. All of the questionnaires were completed with only this child in mind for the duration of the program. This child was also the child who was involved in each of the parent-child activities. Program objectives guided selection of the measures, and the description of program impact that follows is also organized around these objectives. Exclusive reliance upon parent reports does have its drawbacks in terms of concerns about self-serving biases, literacy issues, and method bias when reporting on child behavior—aspects of the parent's personality may color perceptions of the child's behavior. However, direct observations were not practical because of the large sample and distances between sites, the children were too young to report on their parents' behavior, and few of the children were enrolled in preschool programs, which meant that we could not collect teacher reports.

To compensate for these drawbacks, we compared parents' reports of child behavior to data from the DTBY children's program staff at the end of each workshop series and found substantial agreement ($r = .69$). Mothers and fathers also provided similar information about their children ($r = .75$). Finally, we used multiple measures of self-appraisals and child-rearing practices—specific ratings, global ratings, and/or open-ended responses—that generally yielded consistent findings.

Are the Measures Appropriate for Diverse Families?

Literacy and cultural equivalence are significant issues when assessing a multiethnic, low-income population (Knight et al., 1994). Many of the measures we chose for this evaluation had been used successfully with low-income parents who are at risk for abuse or with teenage populations; both groups often function at a sixth-grade reading level or below. However, we used several approaches to determine whether the instruments were appropriate for our target population. First, all instruments were evaluated for readability and had reading levels between grades 4.0 and 6.5. Second, faculty with expertise in adolescence evaluated both the curricular materials and the evaluation instruments for their utility with teenage parents. Similarly, local experts who were familiar with Native American or African-American culture suggested some changes in wording or administration to make items more easily understood. Finally, all evaluation instruments were administered orally to obtain more valid data from participants who had low reading levels.

What Changes Occurred in Parents' Self-Appraisals?

We used the Self-Perceptions of the Parental Role (SPPR; MacPhee, Benson, & Bullock, 1986) to measure parents' feelings of competence and satisfaction with their parental role. One scale on the Parent-Child Relationship Inventory (see later) also measures parental satisfaction. The SPPR has good internal reliabilities and correlates with other measures of self-esteem. Higher levels of self-esteem have been found to relate positively to internal attributions for successful parental performance (MacPhee & Rattenborg, 1991), to caregiving experiences with children (MacPhee et al., 1986), and to levels of social support (MacPhee et al., 1986; Seybold, Fritz & MacPhee, 1991). On the other hand, SPPR scores correlate negatively with levels of stress, difficult child behavior (MacPhee et al., 1986), and the use of inconsistent or harsh disciplinary practices (Fritz & MacPhee, 1991; MacPhee & Rattenborg, 1991).

Parents' feelings of competence (i.e., self-efficacy) and satisfaction both increased significantly between the beginning and end of the workshops (Fig. 6.1). These program effects were sustained through the Year 2 follow-up; the intervention group improved and the control group remaining stable (for details, see Miller-Heyl et al., 1998). Changes in parent self-appraisals were both *consistent* across cohorts and time and *powerful*—large increases relative to those of parents in the nonintervention group ($p < .0001$) (Fig. 6.2.). Open-ended evaluations of the workshops confirmed the importance of these effects. The most liked aspects of the workshops were enhanced self-awareness, self-esteem, or self-confidence.

How Were Changes in Self-Responsibility Measured?

A core goal of this project was to increase parents' internal locus of control, or sense that they can affect what happens to them and their children, and to teach

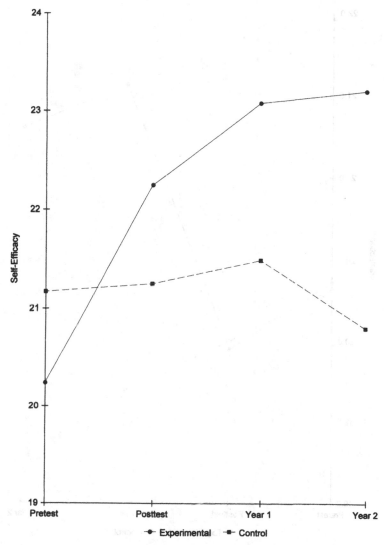

Figure 6.1.   Self-efficacy. Parents increase in self-efficacy.

them to make more accurate causal attributions for behavior. Parents are less likely to set high goals and persist in accomplishing them if they think that chance or luck governs life events, if they blame themselves for their children's negative behavior, or if they see themselves as incompetent parents. Thus, if parents learn that they *do* have control over some aspects of their own lives, including the way their children behave, and if they take credit for successful outcomes, they will

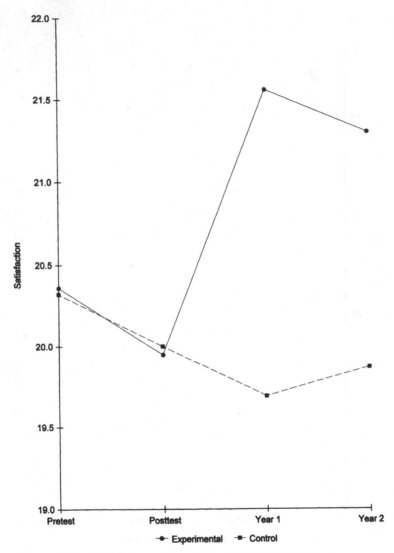

Figure 6.2.   Satisfaction with parenting. Parental satisfaction increases.

become more effective parents and citizens. Two components of self-responsibility were measured: locus of control and causal attributions.

Parents' locus of control was assessed with the IPC scale (Levenson, 1974, 1981), which measures three components of control: (1) Internal control, where people believe that they have control over outcomes; (2) Powerful Others, where others control outcomes; and (3) Chance, where luck or fate determines what happens. Internal and test–retest reliabilities were adequate (.64 to .78). These scales are not correlated with social desirability but they are with fatalism. Finally, measures of self-esteem are strongly, positively related to Internal but negatively correlated with Powerful Others.

Attributions are beliefs about who is responsible for *specific* outcomes in contrast to locus of control, which is a *generalized* expectancy. For example, when asked about the difficulty of getting a child to go to bed, a parent may say that (a) she *Lacks the Ability* to handle the problem, (b) she hasn't made sufficient *Effort* to get the child in bed, (c) it is a difficult *Situation* with which to cope, or (d) it is the child's fault for being so difficult (*Child Blame*). These parent attributions are obviously related to locus of control but are more specific to the everyday problems of being a parent.

The attribution measure consisted of six vignettes that depicted different types of behavior that may be problematic for parents (see Dix & Grusec, 1985; Rosenberg & Reppucci, 1985). Three vignettes concerned violations of moral standards or household rules, and the others were related to oppositional behavior. Then, the respondent rated how applicable four types of causal attribution are as explanations for the parent's difficulty in coping with the child's behavior: lack of ability, task difficulty, insufficient effort, and child blame. This measure is a simplified version of Sirignano and Lachman's (1985) personal control scale. Internal consistencies were adequate in a study of abusive and distressed low-income Colorado parents (MacPhee & Rattenborg, 1991) as well as in the DTBY sample (.76–.88). In terms of validity, parents who know more about child development are less likely to blame the child for difficult behavior. Internal attributions for failure (lack of ability or effort) are also negatively correlated with parental self-esteem (MacPhee & Rattenborg, 1991), and external attributions about the situation are related to external locus of control. However, many parents did not make distinctions among the different types of attributions, and contrary to theory, child-blaming attributions were not related to harsh punishment or to perceptions of the child as more difficult and defiant. One possible reason is that the measure requires abstract, "what if" thinking for parents to put themselves in the situations depicted in the vignettes and to imagine how they would respond.

Did the Program Affect Self-Responsibility?

This is a case where the long-term follow-up showed sleeper effects. The DTBY program seemed to have little impact on the locus of control. Belief in Chance declined significantly in both groups with time, and Native Americans were specially likely to believe in Powerful Others and Chance, but there was no differential effect of the intervention. However, sleeper effects were found on the attribution measure. Few changes were noted until the Year 2 follow-up, except for decreases between the beginning and end of the DTBY workshops on Lack of Ability and Child Blame. Small intervention effects in attributions to effort emerged at the Year 1 follow-up ($p < .05$), and even larger changes were evident at the Year 2 follow-up on all scales except situational attributions (Fig. 6.3). These changes in attributions are consistent with other program effects because decreased self-blaming should accompany increases in self-esteem, and less child blaming may be an important contributor to decreased use of harsh punishment. The sleeper effect may be due to a concerted effort by the program staff to target parents' causal reasoning in the later reinforcing workshops, or it could be the result of parents who reframed their efforts as they succeeded with the child-rearing techniques to which they were exposed in DTBY.

How Were Child-Rearing Practices Measured?

A crucial test of the DTBY family program's impact is whether parents make long-term changes in the way they rear their children, particularly in the areas of effective communication and nurturing rather than punitive discipline. Program impact in the child-rearing domain was assessed with three measures. The Parent-Child Relationship Inventory (PCRI; Gerard, 1994) included three scales related to DTBY objectives: *Limit Setting* or use of consistent control versus coercion and child defiance; *Autonomy*, which concerned encouraging independence versus being permissive and protective; and family *Communication*. Test–retest and alpha reliabilities range from .71 to .92 (Gerard, 1994). Validity has been documented by correlations with other measures of parent self-esteem and child-rearing practices; the PCRI is unrelated to social desirability.

On the second measure, parents reported how often they used each of 12 different disciplinary practices. These were summed into two composites, based on factor analyses (Fritz & MacPhee, 1991; MacPhee & Rattenborg, 1991): *Harsh Punishment*, including spanking, threatening, and criticizing; and *Rational Guidance*, including reasoning, choices, and time-out. The internal reliability of Harsh Punishment is adequate (.81) but is low for Rational Guidance (.64). Parents who felt more competent in the parenting role and who had more prior direct-care experience with children had lower scores on Harsh Punishment and higher scores on Rational Guidance (MacPhee & Rattenborg, 1991). Two studies found significant effects of parent education programs on high-risk parents on Harsh Punishment (Fritz & MacPhee, 1991; MacPhee & Rattenborg, 1991).

The third measure was based on caregivers' open-ended responses to the vignettes: "What would you do or say next in this situation?" Responses were coded into 1 of 21 child-rearing practices, which in turn were assigned a weight from 1 to 5 according to how effective the strategy would be in causing long-term,

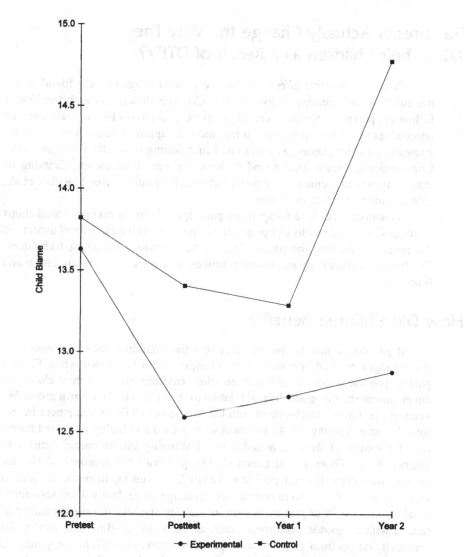

Figure 6.3.   Child blame attributions. Parents reduce child blame.

positive changes in children. Thus, scores on this *Vignettes* measure reflect parents' reasoning and ability to apply what they have learned in DTBY to new circumstances. Interrater agreement was high ($kappa = .51$, $p < .0001$).

Do Parents Actually Change the Way They Raise Their Children as a Result of DTBY?

Consistent positive effects of the intervention program were found on all measures of child rearing (Figs. 6.4 and 6.5). Specifically, through the Year 2 follow-up, parents in the intervention group were much less likely to use punitive approaches and were more likely to respond with appropriate child management strategies on the vignettes, as well as on Limit Setting ($p < .01$). Changes on the Communication scale were found through the Year 1 follow-up. Granting of autonomy, which seems to be strongly influenced by culture (see MacPhee et al., 1996), remained stable over time.

As with changes in self-appraisals, participants' comments on the workshops dovetailed with the results of our questionnaire. One of the most liked aspects of the program was that the parents learned new, positive parenting techniques. The two most commonly mentioned practices were effective communication and time-out.

How Did Children Benefit?

If parents do modify the way they rear their children, then one would expect changes in child behavior. These changes might be of two types. First, if parents provide a more cognitively enriched environment, then their children's development should be accelerated relative to their peers in the control group. We assessed the rate of development with the Minnesota Child Development Inventory (Ireton & Thwing, 1974), the most widely used and highly respected parent report measure of developmental level. Following the recommendations of Sturner, Funk, Thomas, and Green (1982), and with the approval of the test authors, we reduced the item pool from 320 to 75 by omitting items on the General Development scale that were outside our target age range. Internal and test–retest reliabilities were .90 or greater. In terms of validity, the MCDI is significantly correlated with diagnostic instruments such as the Stanford–Binet and Bayley. Its sensitivity ranges from .60 to .80, and specificity from .80 to .97, meaning that it is highly accurate in discriminating between delayed and normal development (see Byrne, Backman, & Smith, 1986; Gottfried, Guerin, Spencer & Meyer, 1984; Guerin & Gottfried, 1987). In terms of utility with various populations, Sturner et al. (1987) used the MCDI for preschool screening in a low-income, largely African-American county in North Carolina. They found that it is significantly

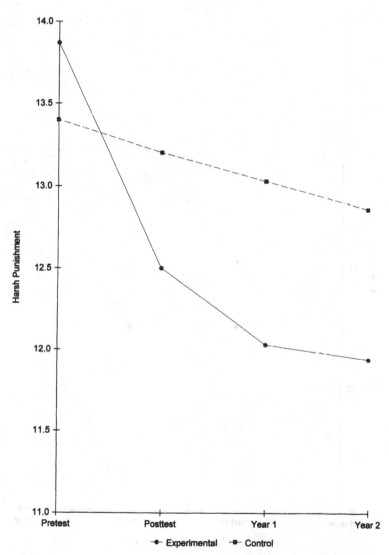

Figure 6.4.   Harsh punishment decreases. Parents decrease harsh punishment.

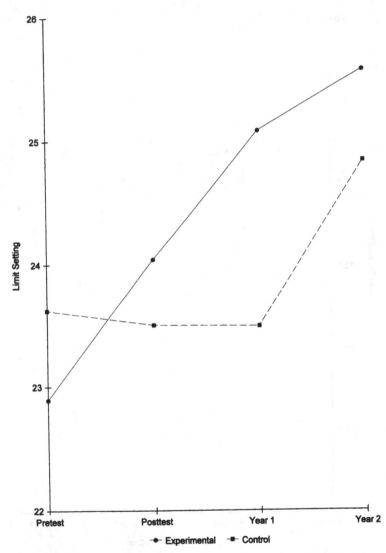

Figure 6.5.   Limit setting increased. Parents increase use of limit setting.

related to longer diagnostic tests, *unless* three or more items are left blank. Such nonresponses may reflect lower reading levels and may be less likely if the inventory is administered orally.

If participants are using more effective methods of controlling their child's behavior, then the parents should report lower levels of difficult child behavior. Difficult behavior in young children may be a warning sign of later aggression and conduct disorders, which are related to substance abuse, delinquency, and school problems. Difficult behavior was assessed with the Behavior Checklist for Infants and Children (MacPhee, 1986), which contains brief descriptions of 42 child behaviors. The caregiver checks how often each one occurs in the target child (frequency) and the degree to which the behavior is problematic. Twelve behaviors represent social competencies. Reliabilities for the Total Problem score exceed .90, indicating that the BCIC is sensitive to individual changes. Correlations between Frequency and Problem scores are high ($r = .75$) for a composite of defiant, aggressive behavior, which is not surprising given that high-intensity noxious behaviors are more likely to be problematic if they are more frequent. Other evidence for validity includes correlations with temperament ratings (or activity level). Problem scores also are inversely related to mothers' feelings of competence and satisfaction with parenthood.

The most striking and consistent findings related to child behavior are the large changes with time. The total number of problem behaviors decreased over the course of the workshops and between pretest and each follow-up, regardless of exposure to the intervention. Such decreases on the BCIC problem score are likely due to maturation, as these children move from the "terrible twos" and threes and approach school age. The effects of intervention did emerge at each follow-up when we looked at a subset of items related to oppositional, defiant behavior (Fig. 6.7). (In a replication project, we found that oppositional behavior and coercive relationships with parents also declined significantly in the intervention group.)

Similarly, increases in developmental level were uniform across all groups and times of measurement (Fig. 6.6). Although normative changes were observed in the control group, children who participated in the DTBY program showed an accelerated pattern of development that was significant at each annual follow-up ($p < .01$). These effects of intervention were particularly evident for the Native American children.

How Did the Intervention Affect Stress and Social Support?

One segment of the DTBY curriculum teaches families stress management techniques. Accordingly, we included the Stress scale from the PCRI; high scores indicate that the parent is overburdened with child-rearing responsibilities and

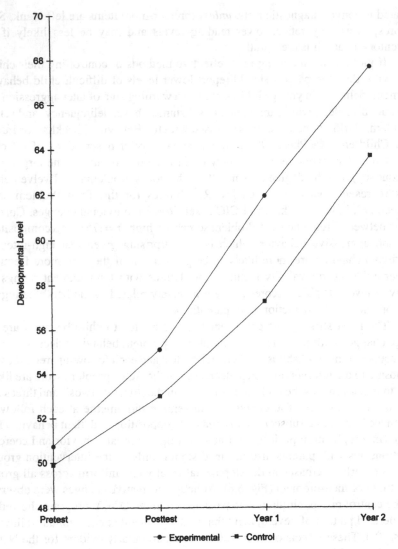

Figure 6.6. Child developmental level. Experimental group shows larger gains.

money worries. In other analyses, we found that this measure is the best single predictor of problematic child-rearing practices. However, the program did not have a discernible effect on parents' stress levels, which may be due to fact that other concepts receive greater emphasis in the curriculum.

The caregivers also completed a measure of social support at baseline and

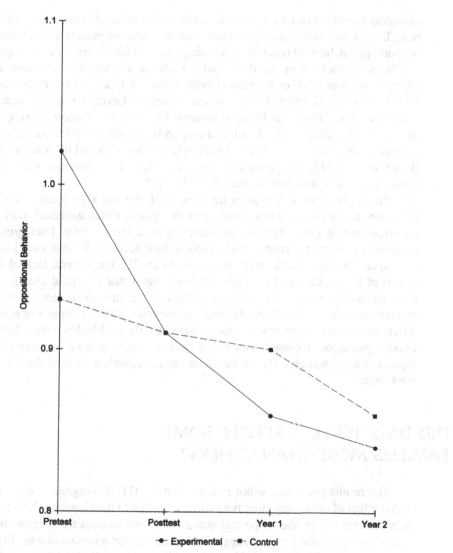

Figure 6.7. Child oppositional behavior. Experimental group decreases opposition.

then yearly thereafter. We measured social support because the workshops focused in part on helping parents to build more effective support systems and parents with higher levels of support were expected to be more capable parents. The Social Network Questionnaire (Antonucci, 1986) measures various dimensions of the parents' social support systems, including network size, perceived closeness to and contact with network members, the types of functions provided (e.g., babysitting, financial help, advice), and how satisfied parents are with their support system. Internal reliabilities are adequate (.80) for our measure of support satisfaction (MacPhee et al., 1996) and are .90 for a composite of emotional support functions in other research (Levitt, Weber, & Clark, 1986). Prior work with low-income children (Levitt, Guacci-Franco, & Levitt, 1993) and parents (MacPhee et al., 1996) has found consistent differences in sources of support among various ethnic groups. Emotional support is typically related to parent self-appraisals (MacPhee et al., 1996), as well as to relationships and life satisfaction (Levitt et al., 1986). The potency of emotional support is consistent with prior research on social networks (Cohen & Wills, 1985).

Briefly, there were four main findings. First, the one significant effect of intervention observed was in satisfaction with support, which increased more in the experimental group than in the control group. Over a year, both groups increased the amount of contact with people in their network. Second, each index of support was quite stable over time (rs = .45 to .71). The general lack of the effects of intervention and the high stability suggest that structural changes in these parents' social systems occur gradually, if at all, although parents' *perceptions* of networks can be reframed through intervention. Third, a number of ethnic differences in social support were observed (for details, see MacPhee et al., 1996). Finally, participant feedback shows that the opportunity to build or strengthen support systems was perceived as one of the more valuable aspects of the DTBY workshops.

DID DARE TO BE YOU HELP SOME FAMILIES MORE THAN OTHERS?

The results presented before indicate that the DTBY program had the intended effect of enhancing effective parenting and child development. However, these findings beg another important question, For whom does the program best work? The "uniformity myth" suggests that intervention approaches and clients are interchangeable (Dance & Neufeld, 1988), yet (some!) therapists, service providers, and evaluators recognize that certain families are at greater risk when they seek intervention services and these services benefit some families more than others. The limited research on this issue is contradictory; some studies find that children and parents from more "deprived" social and economic backgrounds profit the least from intervention programs (Bronfenbrenner, 1975; Johnson & Walker, 1991), whereas others find that prevention programs are most beneficial for the most disadvantaged children (Barnett, 1995).

In the following sections, we discuss three types of individual differences that might moderate the impact of the DTBY program. First, we consider risk factors such as parent age and socioeconomic status. These are often called *social address variables* because they describe the person's social standing ("address") but do not reveal much about actual adjustment and functioning. The second section considers process variables such as parent self-efficacy and stress, which may be the more critical risk factors. Finally, we turn to variations in the way the program was delivered, which involves a look at site variations and measures of implementation.

How Well Does the Program Work for Families Who Vary in Risk?

By design, DTBY is a prevention program that enhances resiliency and provides support rather than crisis intervention or therapy. Thus, individuals with high composite risk scores may not benefit from the program. Yet individuals in the intervention group who had high risk scores did not drop out of the program or fail to benefit. The program evaluators first asked the site coordinators to name parents who, in their estimation, were coping with so many problems that they could not benefit from the program. When the site coordinators reviewed the files of high-risk parents who completed the program and had extreme scores on the risk index, the general consensus was that, despite the odds, they benefited the most from the program. Thus, the DTBY program is appropriate for even very high-risk families, and the social address variables we used in the risk index are not highly correlated with the motivation to change.

Using a more quantitative approach, we identified "types" of parents who varied in their risk profiles to see if certain types benefited more from DTBY. The types were identified by cluster analysis, which grouped parents who were similar in their economic resources and social capital (i.e., age, education, and marital status). Two clusters were relatively advantaged; one ethnically diverse group held mostly blue-collar jobs, whereas the other consisted of middle-class Anglo mothers who worked part time. Another cluster was predominately traditional families that had married homemakers, more children, low stress, and high social support. The remaining two clusters had the highest risk scores; one type consisted of working single mothers and the other tended to be unemployed young mothers. These two groups had the highest levels of welfare dependence (61% and 79%, respectively) and, not surprisingly, the highest levels of stress.

Although these parent types differed from each other at baseline on a number of child-rearing variables, there were very few instances of differential program impact. For instance, regardless of cluster, parents in the intervention group were less inclined to use coercive, punitive practices and became more effective in using democratic control (Limit Setting). Parent type did moderate the program's impact on the measures of autonomy granting and parent self-efficacy. In the two very high-risk clusters, parents in the control group became much worse on these variables, whereas in the intervention group, the highest risk parents improved more than other workshop participants. In contrast, the low-risk, middle-class parents tended to become more confident with time regardless of participation in DTBY. The DTBY program was generally beneficial to all participants but, on a few measures, was especially helpful for the most at-risk families.

Similar results emerged from Wood's (1998) comparison of adolescent and older mothers. She pooled data from three different data sets in which the DTBY family program was provided to diverse, at-risk families. The young mothers had given birth before the age of 18 and were no older than 22 at the time of the baseline assessment, whereas the older mothers had given birth after age 21 and were at least 26 at entry into the program. Although these two groups differed in many respects on the parenting variables, especially stress, they showed similar patterns of improvement as a result of the DTBY program.

Does the Program Affect Family Processes?

Social risk variables only weakly predict which parents benefit the most from the DTBY program. An alternative is to focus on their actual functioning as parents. Guided by our impact theory and by process models of child rearing (Belsky, 1984), we honed in on three variables that are consistently related to capable child rearing: parent self-efficacy, emotionally supportive social networks, and stress.

At baseline in this project (and in later replications), parents who have poor self-appraisals are much more likely to rely upon harsh punishment, to rate their children's behavior as more problematic, to blame their child for parenting difficulties, and to get angrier at child misdeeds. This recipe for child abuse is found regardless of the degree of psychosocial risk or ethnicity (see MacPhee et al., 1996). Turning to social support, parents who are less satisfied with their levels of social support are less confident as parents, blame themselves and their child for parenting problems, perceive that their children are more difficult, and are more coercive in their child-rearing practices. Finally, parents who report being under more stress are less satisfied with the parental role, make self-denigrating attributions, are angrier at child misbehavior, and are involved in more coercive, punitive relationships with their children. The latter profile is consistent with the way in which depressed parents function (Gelfand & Teti, 1990; Goodman & Gotlib, 1999). These correlations support the wisdom of focusing on empowering parents, fostering strong social networks, and increasing their stress management skills.

Do these process variables relate to how much parents benefit from DTBY? Changes in self-perceived competence seem to be an important but not necessary condition for improved child-rearing practices. Miller-Heyl et al. (1998) reported that parents who showed the largest increases in parent self-efficacy also showed the greatest improvements in democratic control, were the least likely to use harsh punishment at the Year 1 follow-up (even though they were the most punitive at baseline), and changed the most in their ratings of difficult child behavior. These results held even after taking initial levels of functioning and risk into account. The caveat here is that parents whose self-efficacy remained stable still showed some improvement, albeit modest, in their child-rearing practices. Even so, our analyses of the pretest data and results of the intervention strongly suggest that programs designed to enhance parents' resilience should include a component that targets social–cognitive processes. Parents' perceptions of themselves and their children are part and parcel of skilled child rearing. This recommendation stands in contrast to that of some critics who have argued that an emphasis upon self-esteem in family intervention does more harm than good, at least compared to a "rightful" focus on family processes (Burr & Christensen, 1992).

Improved social support was not as central to changes in child rearing. Although the DTBY program resulted in greater satisfaction with support and parents valued the opportunity to strengthen their networks, this variable at baseline did not predict differential effects of the intervention in either the original trial or the replication. Still, it may be an essential program component when geographical isolation is an issue or when parents do not have extended families to help with child rearing.

Like self-efficacy, stress seems to be a critical moderator of program impact. In two different intervention trials with DTBY, we found that initial levels of stress were modestly related to changes in self-blaming attributions and anger, and strongly correlated with changes in effective child-rearing practices. Identical findings emerged when we used a measure of coercive interactions between parent and child. In all cases, the more parents were at risk, the more they improved in terms of anger control, less harsh punishment, setting appropriate limits, and more open communication.

In conclusion, although DTBY is effective with the majority of families, it is particularly beneficial for parents who are at high risk for maltreatment because of low self-efficacy, high stress, and coercive relationships with their children. These results suggest that DTBY should have a favorable cost/benefit ratio given the expense of involvement with child protection services. Our findings also imply that in secondary or indicated prevention programs, screening for risk should focus on process variables rather than static social address variables.

Do Variations in Implementation Alter Program Benefits?

The way in which a program is implemented may also affect how much individual participants benefit from it. In the first demonstration project, we had rather limited information on program implementation, but we had a wealth of data in the replication trial. As it turns out, there were few instances in which implementation mattered.

- The only site difference in program impact was on the measure of developmental level. In both the original and replication trials, Native American children showed larger gains on the MCDI than children at the other sites. We find the general lack of site differences remarkable because the risk profiles and ethnic composition varied markedly across sites, and the implementation logbooks documented pervasive differences in how much emphasis was placed on different curriculum modules.

- Perceptions of the program were not related to impact. One might expect that parents who are more satisfied with their experiences in DTBY would also have gained more from the program. Although the vast majority of parents were quite pleased with the program, a few did have ratings below midpoint on the client satisfaction items. These mildly critical parents tended to be poorer, more stressed, more punitive, and less satisfied with the parental role. Yet posttest perceptions of the program were unrelated to how much parents improved. Program facilitators might draw the lesson that even when parents whine about the program, there's still a good chance that they are gaining something from the experience; their complaints may have more to do with background stress.

- In both the original and replication projects, facilitators completed detailed implementation logbooks that recorded which activities were used, how activities were modified, how much time was spent on-task as opposed to on personal issues, and how engaged the participants were in the group process. Aspects of group cohesion and openness to new ideas were somewhat related to differential change but, by and large, none of the 40 implementation variables predicted how much participants would benefit from DTBY.

- More traditional Hispanic and Native American parents may differ from acculturated parents in their child-rearing practices, and they may be less receptive to intervention materials that are based on an "Anglo model" that emphasizes communication and democratic child rearing. An acculturation scale was included in the replication trial to test this hypothesis. Even though acculturation was correlated with autonomy and reasoning at baseline, it was unrelated to the degree of change on the various parenting measures. The degree of acculturation did not influence the amount that families benefited.

Clearly, the DTBY curriculum is robust with respect to variations in the way it is implemented. The program resulted in similar benefits to families despite variations in participant risk and culture, in community ecology, and in facilitators' styles. We attribute these main effects of the program to a clearly articulated theory of change—which means that all facilitators and parents know what the program's objectives are—and to careful selection and training of the staff who implements the curriculum. It also helps that the staff is strict in applying the incentives so that all participants receive at least 20 hours of the program.

DO INTERVENTIONISTS AND EVALUATORS MAKE STRANGE BEDFELLOWS?

We end this chapter with a few musings on the collaboration between the intervention staff, which put DTBY principles into practice, and the program evaluators, who are charged with documenting the implementation and impact of the program. This relationship can be fraught with misunderstanding, mistrust, and even loathing. In our case, though, the intervention staff and the evaluators maintained a working partnership for close to 15 years. Why?

One essential reason that this partnership has worked well is that the program staff and evaluators have a compatible theoretical orientation regarding family functioning and what constitutes effective prevention. The evaluators were steeped in ecological, systems, and social–cognitive theory before their involvement with DTBY, and through hands-on work in prevention, the intervention staff understood the importance of community context, nested systems, and self-efficacy. Regardless of their role in the program, all staff members strongly believe in the importance of early prevention that builds on family strengths and enhances resiliency factors, and in the necessity of attending to human diversity.[1] These common assumptions about ways to effect change and which risk and resiliency mechanisms to target, meant that all staff members could make meaningful suggestions about effective intervention strategies and about evaluation procedures that were consistent with the program's philosophy. As Kurt Lewin said, there is nothing so practical as a good theory.

The interventionists and evaluators also have mutual respect for each other's competence and dedication. The interventionists have a very good sense of the problems that families face in the real world, the way these issues affect program implementation, and the practicalities of collecting evaluative data. This utilitarian perspective resulted in a number of good suggestions for how the data should be collected, ways to administer measures, and ways to minimize attrition. The evaluators' content expertise, in turn, led to suggestions for curricular activities, ways to make the curriculum developmentally appropriate, and ways to conduct

---

[1]MacPhee, D., Kreutzer, J. C., & Fritz, J. (1994). Infusing a multicultural perspective into human development courses. *Child Development, 65,* 699–715.
MacPhee, D., Oltjenbruns, K. A., Fritz, J. J., & Kreutzer, J. C. (1994). Strategies for infusing curricula with a multicultural perspective. *Innovative Higher Education, 18,* 289–309.

effective parent education classes. The intervention staff also learned a bit—perhaps more than they cared to know—about assessment, research design, theories of human development, and statistics.

We did find that our roles blurred at times. Collaborative problem solving was the rule at retreats, which meant that the evaluators might have input on the curriculum and the intervention staff would suggest changes in the evaluation procedures. Such collaboration was made easier because interventionists and evaluators alike were open to learning and were willing to teach each other. On the other hand, this blurring of roles could be problematic. At times, the evaluators found it difficult to maintain a stance of scientific objectivity when it became clear that DTBY was having a powerful impact on families. We had to remind ourselves that we were reporters, not advocates. The intervention staff was also involved in collecting evaluation data. This dual role can be quite difficult because the program staff views its relationships with families through the lens of support and advocacy, which is contrary to the need for even-handed objectivity when collecting data. In later replications, the staff was divided into two groups: those involved in data collection and those involved in service delivery. This may not always be possible, but a clarity in the purpose of each role helps to specify staff behavior in its different activities.

There is an inherent tension, widely acknowledged in human services programs, between expenditures on direct services to at-risk families versus devoting limited resources to rigorous evaluation. This tension arises because service providers prefer to help those with the greatest needs, as opposed to randomly assigning individuals to an intervention group, and they question the ethics of withholding help from a no-treatment control group. Yet random assignment to intervention and control groups is the only means to determine whether a program *caused* changes in behavior. In most respects, this tension was successfully negotiated in the DTBY project, except for a decision to allow families to switch groups after the Year 1 follow-up. More families than anticipated made this choice resulting in a significant loss of control participants at the San Luis Valley site, and compromised the ability to detect long-term site variations in program impact. The lesson we learned from this experience was to restrict the number of control families who could later enroll in the intervention group and to assign them by lottery.

Finally, our partnership was successful for pragmatic reasons and for personal reasons. Pragmatically, a program staff needs evaluators to assess how services are being provided and to determine whether the services are making a difference. What might be overlooked in this one-sided account is that the DTBY evaluators also needed a way to field test postulates about the importance of social–cognitive processes to effective parenting, about cultural variations in child rearing and social networks, and so forth. On a personal level, virtually all of the staff members are optimistic folks and enjoy each other's company. This alone has made the work a real pleasure.

What Activities Enhance this Relationship?

A key activity that contributed to the successful working relationship between the evaluation and program staffs was a yearly miniconference. This retreat-like two- to three-day activity was attended by all of the staff from both the evaluation and program delivery components. The playing field was level. Objectives that had been reached and those still to be attained were outlined. Accomplishments were celebrated. Difficulties from both "sides" were open for mutual troubleshooting and problem solving. This process led to an inside view of the challenges that faced both the program and evaluation staffs. The miniconference was conducted by following the same principles that guide the rest of the program. The successful working relationships developed add credence to the validity of the DTBY model.

What Add/Aides Enhance this Relationship?

How Can a Community or Agency Determine If It Can Successfully Implement the DARE to be You Program?

ASSESSING THE RESOURCES NECESSARY TO IMPLEMENT THE PROGRAM

What makes a program work at one site but not at another? The reasons can be elusive, but several factors optimize the chances for success. Some are so important that if they are not present, the project is likely to fail. These factors are common across many programs (see Schorr, 1989), but we will focus on lessons learned from implementing DTBY in a number of communities.

WHO IS INVOLVED IN THE PROGRAM?

The Sponsoring Agency or Organization

One sure path to failure occurs when an agency or organization takes on the program with less than a full commitment to make it work for families in their community. Why might a sponsor make a half-hearted investment? DTBY is viewed as a fundable program, so that an agency might apply for the money believing that the program can simply be added to the responsibilities of an already overworked staff. It won't work. Does the board of directors support DTBY's concepts? If a key stakeholder on the board or in a collaborating agency is lukewarm or hostile to DTBY's approach, the prospects for success are dim. An administrator may be attracted to the program philosophy or approach but does not have the buy-in and commitment from the staff. In that case, it is rare that the program would be implemented effectively. A staff person believes it will work for families in the community but does not have the functional support from administration. It will die on the vine. If there is no one person in the organization who has time and influence and is passionate about the program concept, it will sputter.

What if the agency does not have space for the staff? The staff should be housed within the agency for several essential reasons. First, if it is not on site, it conveys the message that the program is not as important as other programs—because space is not made available. Second, physical distance creates barriers to communication with other agency staff. Staff supervision and training are more difficult. Other staff members often become resentful because a trainer just pops in, "makes demands and messes," and leaves. Even when the staff members prefer to work at home, they should be encouraged to prepare for their classes on-site because it enhances communication and team building. DTBY is more staff and resource intensive and has more space requirements than many programs, so that the entire sponsoring agency should be informed about program events. The program staff often needs to make an extra effort to maintain good communication with the rest of the agency.

The sponsor should be credible with other agencies in the community, with individuals who control access to necessary resources (including target popula-tions), and with the families who will be served. Specifically, the sponsoring agency must be connected in positive ways to other community agencies that work with families. A key test for community connections might be that the potential program director can call four or five key agencies in the community, explain the DTBY concept, and be able to put together a steering committee or advisory group with letters of commitment for referrals or contributed services. If sponsors cannot do this, then they might not have sufficient community support to implement the program.

Agency credibility is also manifest if target families already walk in the door and if families generally perceive that the agency is supportive and effective. Such demand for services is a boost in reaching populations of high-risk families. If the target population does not already use the sponsor's services, can the agency collaborate with another site to hold family classes at a place that is accessed and perceived as welcoming? An example would be our Native American site. Fami-lies from this site rarely walked in the door of the DTBY offices in Cortez when the program started. In part, this was due to distance because most of the families live 15 miles away from Cortez. It was also because we had not previously been a "service" agency. However, we arranged for the family classes to be held in the tribal community at the Head Start facility, which families did frequent. The classes were held there, and the Head Start faculty also played a key role in recruiting families into DTBY.

The literature on community mental health and prevention programs yields several important barriers to access that agencies should consider before implementing DTBY (see Schorr, 1989). One of the more important obstacles is inconvenient location and times. If the program is offered when few families can attend, and especially if transportation to the site is not available, families will not enroll (Northam, 1996; Owens, 1994; Soderlund, Epstein, Quinn, Cumblad, & Petersen, 1995). Access is critical in the early stages of a program before it becomes visible and builds a solid reputation. After the program and staff are known and respected, we have found that families will drive an hour or more, use their bicycles, or even hitchhike to attend workshops. Lack of child care is an important barrier for many parenting programs (Kelley, Perloff, Morris, & Liu, 1992), which is one reason why DTBY's two-generational approach is effective. The cost of getting to class can be an impediment (Kauffman & Poulin, 1994; Soderlund et al., 1995), especially for minority families (Woodward, Dwinell, & Arons, 1992), which reinforces the importance of providing monetary incentives. Therefore, if an agency cannot locate a convenient place or schedule classes when families can attend, the agency may not be able to replicate the program.

Key Staff

Staff selection and training also can reduce some barriers. Research on community health care has found that provider/client rapport is critical in preventing client dropout (Kazdin, Holland, & Crowley, 1997). Such rapport can be fostered in an individual case management model, so that families meet with the same provider over time (Schorr, 1989), and by training providers in effective, client-centered communication. Yet, many clients in the mental health system perceive that providers are rude and insensitive, and many service providers perceive that low-income clients are unmotivated and deficient (Judd & Forgues, 1989). Such attitudes breed suspicion and victim blaming and obviously interfere with effective interventions. Finally, Spanish-speaking clients report that one of the greatest obstacles to receiving services is that the staff cannot speak their language (DeGagni, Wietlisbach, Poisson, Stein, & Royeen, 1994; Northam, 1996). Each of these barriers can be surmounted by thoroughly planning services and carefully selecting the staff. For example, Kauffman and Poulin (1994) found that potential clients were more likely to seek services if they perceived that the program is effective.

Lack of commitment to the program can be shown by an unwillingness to find and train capable program staff. As Slaughter (1988) noted, "The most well-designed family services programs may fail without suitable and enthusiastic people responsible for their administration and implementation" (p. 469). Another critical component is nurturing the staff's commitment to work together.

Team Building

The team that works with families is the key to the program's success. This includes the parent trainer, the child program coordinator, evaluators (if appropriate), teen educators, and other support staff. If this team cannot meet together regularly, it will undermine the program's success—in the way the program is implemented and also in the sense of teamwork and purpose, as well as support for the families. If several of the key staff just arrive "at the bell," do their parts, and leave without being involved in either planning or postsession team meetings, the program will be less effective. An agency that does not provide funds for team meetings is likely to have to cope with inconsistent programming and potential failure.

Staff Qualifications

Because of the program's emphasis on fostering personal strengths and promoting personal efficacy, the most effective staff members are those who already demonstrate personal and teaching efficacy, who are nonjudgmental and accepting, and who can look for the positive attributes of families. These traits are among those Slaughter (1988) identified as key for staff members who work with diverse clients in family support programs. For instance, the staff should model control of one's life. A sense of personal agency is associated with successful service delivery. Self-respect and enthusiasm also are critical, as well as "a genuine commitment and camaraderie among workers with a shared mission" (p. 469). The DTBY program will not be as successful if the people who staff it prefer to lecture, are prone to find fault, or promote a personal agenda for parenting that is at odds with prevailing cultural norms. We know of no personnel screening tool for dogmatism and optimism, but such traits are certainly relevant to whether DTBY is successful.

Programs are also more effective if the curricular philosophy is compatible with service providers' goals and their personal philosophies of child rearing and family life (Slaughter, 1988). In our experience, problems in this area might occur when, for example, a parent facilitator views the workshop setting as an opportunity to conduct group therapy rather than to promote resiliency skills. Garbarino (1992) provided another example when he noted that, "One of the greatest obstacles [to providing effective services] is that 'we' need to help 'them'" (p. 260). Instead, staff members need to approach their task as consultants and advocates. Thus, program administrators should take care to assess potential facilitators' views on why people are resilient, on family strengths, and what the "proper" role of a facilitator is in a prevention program that works with high-risk families.

Will the agency work with a target population that is culturally different from their staff or from their usual clients? If so, then trainers should be selected who speak the language and understand the culture. There may be cases where "non-enmeshed outsiders" are actually more effective because they are not immersed in local community politics or long-standing family feuds. One of our sites actually requested that the existing program staff continue training because of their neutrality in the community. In such cases, the agency needs to find out from reliable sources within the target community whether the identified program staff is credible and accepted by the families who will be enrolled or by key local people. Is there someone who can appropriately enact cultural adaptations to the curriculum? If not, the agency probably is not prepared to provide the program.

Training

Many people are qualified to facilitate various parent education and support groups. The following guideline is not intended to question the experience and abilities of potential facilitators. However, if an agency is unwilling to sponsor and have a significant number of future DTBY team members and other staff (including supervisors) attend a training workshop with people who have already implemented the curriculum, the agency is not prepared to deliver the program. This level of commitment is essential for interagency awareness of the program and communication among the staff about the program.

Does anyone on the staff of the sponsoring agency have a formal background in human development, family systems, research-based knowledge of effective parenting practices, child psychology, or closely related fields? There should be internal support for the knowledge base of the program. If not, there should be collaborative support from a partner agency. Without these, the agency may struggle to transmit DTBY's basic concepts to families, even with training or material support. As Slaughter (1988) and others have noted, participants are more likely to invest in the program if they understand the program's goals. Participants trust facilitators more when they discern a congruence between program goals and activities and when they see concrete evidence that they are becoming more skilled parents.

Is the agency willing to staff the children's program to meet the recommended child-to-teacher ratio of 5:1? Is the agency willing to recruit, screen, train, and supervise teen teachers or family class graduates as part of the teaching staff? Is the agency willing to pay for the services of these paraprofessionals instead of depending on volunteers? If the sponsoring agency is not willing to invest in these teaching resources, then it might not be ready to implement the program as designed. As Schorr (1989) found, one way to ruin a successful program is to dilute the intensity of the services or the competence of the staff.

Basic Program Resources

Programs such as DTBY also must have adequate physical and financial resources. For instance, agencies that do not agree philosophically with offering incentives for participation should not implement the program. If an agency views the incentives as important but does not have the will or ability to raise funds for them, it will not be replicating the program with fidelity. Nor will the program be replicated if weekly incentives are provided instead of providing a lump sum upon completion of the program. (One is likely to find much higher attrition rates and more sporadic attendance.) An agency must agree with the philosophy behind the incentives, have the will and means to provide them, and be able to defend them to other community organizations and funders.

We should note that there is nothing magical about a $200 incentive for completing the program. This amount is not based on systematic research to determine what minimum amount is necessary to attract high-risk families to the program and keep them enrolled until the program activities and rapport with staff have them "hooked." Replicating programs could provide valuable information to the field by examining variations in incentives as related to who enrolls (risk profiles are likely to vary with the amount of incentive) and how attrition is affected.

Potential replicators should not assume that it will be easy to find appropriate space in their communities for the program. Especially in small rural communities, the sponsoring agency should find a compatible site before initiating the program and have a commitment (e.g., a letter of agreement) that the space will be available for the full course of the program. Having an alternate space also is recommended. Sponsors can change their minds about hosting the program if something happens that is blamed on the classes: rooms are left messy, items are broken, the janitor complains, or something disappears or is misplaced. Space requirements include a place to serve meals; rooms for adults, infants, toddlers, and older siblings; and one room that is large enough for a parent-child activity. Storage space is also important, or the staff has to transport all of the supplies for meals and workshops each week. Families and staff are annoyed by facilities that are cold, echo-y, or cramped.

The same forethought is important when providing meals. An agency needs to have its ducks in a row as to who will prepare the meals, their cost and quality, and how dependable the food providers will be. All of the sites that have implemented DTBY have horror stories about meals, such as finding glass in the food, poor quality, and not having it ready on time. Petty as they seem, these small factors set the tone for a program, particularly because the family meal is typically the first event at each session. Can the staff buy the materials it needs for the program? Is storage for the materials available at the facility? Does the agency have an agreement with the staff members that they will transport materials each week if necessary, set them up, clean up the site, and arrange for the food? Problems with any of these logistics undermine the program's success in the long run.

Key Program Components

This monograph identified the key program components necessary to replicate the DTBY program for families of preschool youth. If an agency departs from DTBY's conceptual basis by too much or is unwilling to implement its key processes, then it will not be a replication. For instance, if the staff decides to put decision-making activities first and omit the self-efficacy component, the resulting intervention would not be DTBY. The agency might be better served by selecting a model that more closely meets its focus on decision making.

When the required 20 hours of workshops were compressed into a one-shot weekend retreat, the program was not effective, probably because parents had no time to practice skills and reflect on what they were learning. Some programs have excised selected components from the DTBY parent curriculum and offered them in a 6-week series, but this approach also resulted in minimal benefits. Thus, an agency should commit 10 to 12 weeks to each program series. If schedules do not allow for at least a 10-week series, the agency should consider using a different program that might be more narrowly focused and shorter. The effectiveness of DTBY in altering family patterns and enhancing resiliency depends on gradual increases in self-efficacy, building trust, learning how to apply problem-solving techniques, and practicing parenting skills.

Evaluation

With successive replications, the potency of an intervention often grows weaker. Likely explanations include shortcuts in staff training, diminished resources (Schorr, 1989), and especially "program drift" or poorer adherence to the original program model (McGrew, Bond, Dietzen, & Salyers, 1994). Further, when treatment fidelity is not monitored, program drift is more likely to occur (Henggeler, Melton, Brondino, Schere, & Hanley, 1997). For these reasons, we believe that replications of DTBY should commit resources to evaluating program implementation and impact. Doing so will help the program to monitor its effectiveness, and deviations from the DTBY model can be identified as possible explanations for diluted impact. But conducting such evaluative activities, even a scaled-down version of the one we used, requires that someone be available to design and monitor data collection procedures, analyze the data, and monitor fidelity to the program model. If these basic elements are not available, the agency may not be ready to conduct the program.

Follow-Up and Continuation

Does the agency have a way to maintain support for the families after the initial funding runs out? This can take many forms, including support groups, additional classes as the children reach different developmental stages, or a person to call with questions. Referrals to support groups and persons in collaborating agencies might also be considered. An agency must be willing to support families' long-term well-being.

THE BOTTOM LINE

Because of the intensive nature of the DTBY program, agencies should be able to demonstrate commitment to the program at all levels. Agencies have a high probability of success when they are willing to (a) hire an appropriate staff and give it sufficient time and support, (b) provide the space and ancillary resources, (c) give technical support for evaluation activities, and (d) network DTBY facilitators with other staff and the community. Perhaps the core requirement is that someone on the staff is passionate about the program. The more of these factors an agency can bring to bear on issues that face high-risk families, the more likely it is that these families will become resilient and competent.

Conclusion

As important as it is and as reasonable as it may seem, implementing a program that incorporates ecological, human development, and prevention theories is extraordinarily difficult to execute. The invisible reefs and navigational challenges we face include changing political currents that flow in different directions from year to year, and the flotsam are often children. Resources ebb and flow erratically. Community groups often pursue popular or short-term solutions to stay afloat. As a society, we keep our eyes on the near horizon. We find it hard to commit the long-term, substantial resources that may entail sacrifices of turf necessary to steer through the shoals.

We have a solid research base that gives us direction. That base tells us that reducing risks and building resilient, fully functioning youth is not simple. It will not happen in two hours or two days or even two years. It may take a lifetime. It will not happen by modifying only one aspect of a complex developmental process. It requires work with multiple processes across several ecological contexts. One parent or one community agency can make a difference for some individuals. But our society must commit to greater collaboration among systems, and we must invest the consistent resources to prevention strategies that actually make a difference in the lives of families and youth.

Programs that foster the human potential of youth and thus their resilience must be planned from infancy to adulthood. They must cross the boundaries of agencies and microsystems. They must promote age-appropriate competencies of the sort that protect youth from later problems, for we know that such competencies build on each other but may be different at one time in life than another.

In this twenty-first century, we have both a unique opportunity and a challenge. We have passed through a time when our society was divided into three major components: our civil society in which we interacted together in many social, spiritual and community contexts; our capitalistic society in which we are usually employed or are consumers; and our governmental society. At the beginning of the twenty-first century, our civil society is being squeezed out as the other two components grow. This shrinking can be noticed by the smaller attendance at religious organizations, community groups, and the settings where families and communities traditionally interacted to structure and maintain our cultures. Families are caught in the squeeze. Many youth are spending their free time in the streets or in the malls. What cultural values do they learn there? Can we create new ways to restore civil society? Perhaps we have an opportunity to recreate this special place through family-based workshops and organizations.

Beacons directing us to effective prevention exist. Our leaders and citizens must be encouraged to heed them if our youth are to benefit.

References

Antonucci, T. C. (1986). Social support networks: A hierarchical mapping technique. *Generations*, *10*(2), 10–12.

Ashton, P. T., & Webb, R. B. (1986). *Making a difference: Teacher's sense of efficacy and student achievement*. New York: Longman.

Azar, S. T. (1997). A cognitive behavioral approach to understanding and treating parents who physically abuse their children. In D. A. Wolfe et al. (Eds.), *Child abuse: New directions in prevention and treatment across the lifespan* (pp. 79–101). Thousand Oaks, CA: Sage.

Bandura, A. (1986). *Social foundations of thought and action: A social cognitive theory*. Englewood Cliffs, NJ: Prentice-Hall.

Bandura, A. (1997). *Self-efficacy: The exercise of control*. New York: Freeman.

Barnett, W. S. (1995). Long-term effects of early childhood programs on cognitive and school outcomes. *The Future of Children*, *5*(3), 25–30.

Battistich, V., Solomon, D., Watson, M., & Schaps, E. (1997). Caring school communities. *Educational Psychologist*, *32*, 137–151.

Bauman, L. J., Stein, R. E. K., & Ireys, H. T. (1991). Reinventing fidelity: The transfer of social technology among settings. *American Journal of Community Psychology*, *19*, 619–639.

Baumrind, D. (1996). The discipline controversy revisited. *Family Relations*, *45*, 405–414.

Belsky, J. (1984). The determinants of parenting: A process model. *Child Development*, *55*, 83–96.

Benson, P. L., Leffert, N., Scales, P. C., & Blyth, D. A. (1998). Beyond the "village" rhetoric: Creating healthy communities for children and adolescents. *Applied Developmental Science*, *2*, 138–159.

Berkowitz, M. W., & Gibbs, J. C. (1983). Measuring the developmental features of moral discussion. *Merrill-Palmer Quarterly*, *29*, 399–410.

Bierman, K. L., & Greenberg, M. T. (1996). Social skills training in the FAST Track Program. In R. DeV. Peters & R. J. McMahon (Eds.), *Preventing childhood disorders, substance abuse, and delinquency* (pp. 65–89). Thousand Oaks, CA: Sage.

Blakely, C. H., Mayer, J. P., Gottschalk, R. G., Schmitt, N., Davidson, W. S., Roitman, D. B., &

Emshoff, J. G. (1987). The fidelity-adaptation debate: Implications for the implementation of public sector social programs. *American Journal of Community Psychology, 15*, 253–268.

Blechman, E. A. (1991). Effective communication: Enabling multiproblem families to change. In P. A. Cowan & M. Hetherington (Eds.), *Family transitions* (pp. 219–244). Hillsdale, NJ: Erlbaum.

Bloomquist, M. L., August, G. J., Bromback, M. M., Anderson, D. L., & Skare, S. S. (1996). Maternal facilitation of children's problem solving: Relation to disruptive child behavior and maternal characteristics. *Journal of Clinical Child Psychology, 25*, 308–316.

Brody, G. H., Flor, D. L., & Gibson, N. M. (1999). Linking maternal self-efficacy beliefs, developmental goals, parenting practices, and child competence in rural single-parent African-American families. *Child Development, 70*, 1197–1208.

Bronfenbrenner, U. (1975). Is early intervention effective? In U. Bronfenbrenner (Ed.), *Influences on human development* (2nd ed., pp. 329–354). Hinsdale, IL: Dryden.

Bronfenbrenner, U. (1979). *The ecology of human development.* Cambridge, MA: Harvard University.

Bronfenbrenner, U., & Morris, P. A. (1998). The ecology of developmental processes. In W. Damon (Series Ed.) and R. M. Lerner (Vol. Ed.), *Handbook of child psychology,* 5th ed., *Vol. 1, Theoretical models of human development* (pp. 993–1028). New York: Wiley.

Brook, J. S., Brook, D. W., Gordon, A. S., Whiteman, M. L., & Cohen, P. (1986). Some models and mechanisms for explaining the input of maternal and adolescent characteristics on adolescent stage of drug use. *Adolescent Psychology, 22*, 460–467.

Brook, J. S., Brook, D. W., Gordon, A. S., Whiteman, M. L., & Cohen, P. (1990). The psycholosocial etiology of adolescent drug use: A family interactional approach. *Genetic, Social and General Psychology Monographs, 116*, 111–267.

Brounstein, P., & Zweig, J. M. (1999). *Understanding substance abuse prevention: Toward the 21st century. A primer on effective programs* (DHHS Publication No. SMA 99-3301). Rockville, MD: Substance Abuse and Mental Health Administration, Dept. of Health and Human Services.

Brownfield, D., & Sorenson, A. M. (1991). Religion and drug use among adolescents: A social support conceptualization and interpretation. *Deviant Behavior, 12*, 259–276.

Bryk, A. S., & Driscoll, M. E. (1988). *The high school as community: Contextual influences and consequences for students and teachers.* (ERIC Document Reproduction Service No. ED302539)

Bugental, D. B. (1992). Affective and cognitive processes within threat-oriented family systems. In I. E. Sigel, A. V. McGillicuddy-DeLisi, & J. J. Goodnow (Eds.), *Parental belief systems* (pp. 219–248). Hillsdale, NJ: Erlbaum.

Burnett, P. C. (1996). An investigation of the social learning and symbolic interaction models for the development of self-concepts and self-esteem. *Journal of Family Studies, 2*, 57–64.

Burr, W. R., & Christensen, C. (1992). Undesirable side effects of enhancing self-esteem. *Family Relations, 41*, 460–464.

Busch-Rossnagel, N. A., Knauf-Jensen, D. E., & DesRosiers, F. S. (1995). Mothers and others: The role of the socializing environment in the development of mastery motivation. In R. H. MacTurk & G. A. Morgan (Eds.), *Mastery motivation: Origins, conceptualizations, and applications* (pp. 117–145). Norwood, NJ: Ablex.

Bush, P. J., & Iannotti, R. J. (1985). The development of children's health orientation and behaviors: Lessons for substance use. *National Institute on Drug Abuse: Research, Monograph Series No. 56*, 45–74.

Byrne, J. M., Backman, J. E., & Smith, I. M. (1986). Developmental assessment: the clinical use and validity of parental report. *Journal of Pediatric Psychology, 11*, 549–559.

Caplan, N., Whitmore, J. W., & Choy, M. H. (1989). *The boat people and achievement in America: A study of family life, hard work, and cultural values.* Ann Arbor, MI: University of Michigan Press.

Clark, R. D., & Shields, G. (1997). Family communication and delinquency. *Adolescence, 32*, 81–92.

Cochran, M., Larner, M., Riley, D., Gunnarsson, L., & Henderson, C. R. (1990). *Extending families: The social networks of parents and their children.* Cambridge, England: Cambridge University Press.

Cohen, S., & Wills, T. A. (1985). Stress, social support, and the buffering hypothesis. *Psychological Bulletin, 98*, 310–357.

Coie, J. D., & Dodge, K. A. (1998). Aggression and antisocial behavior. In W. Damon (Series Ed.) & N. Eisenberg (Vol. Ed.), *Handbook of child psychology*, 5th ed., *Vol. 3, Social, emotional, and personality development* (pp. 779–862). New York: Wiley

Coie, J. D., Watt, N. F., West, S. G., Hawkins, J. D., Asarnow, J. R., Markman, H. J., Ramey, S. L., Shure, M. B., & Long, B. (1993). The science of prevention: A conceptual framework and some directions for a national research program. *American Psychologist, 48*, 1013–1022.

Comer, J. (1980). *School power*. New York: Free Press.

Connell, J. P., & Ilardi, B. C. (1987). Self-system concomitants of discrepancies between children's and teachers' evaluations of academic competence. *Child Development, 58*, 1297–1307.

Connell, J. P., & Wellborn, J. G. (1991). Competence, autonomy, and relatedness: A motivational analysis of self-system processes. In M. R. Gunnar, L. A. Sroufe, et al. (Eds.), *Self processes and development. The Minnesota Symposium on Child Development* (Vol. 23, pp. 43–77). Hillsdale, NJ: Erlbaum.

Connors, L. J., & Epstein, J. L. (1995). Parent and school partnerships. In M. H. Bornstein (Ed.), *Handbook of parenting. Vol. 4. Applied and practical parenting* (pp. 437–458). Mahwah, NJ: Erlbaum.

Cooley, M. L., & Unger, D. G. (1991). The role of family support in determining developmental outcomes in children of teen mothers. *Child Psychiatry and Human Development, 21*, 217–234.

Coombs, R. H., & Landsverk, J. (1988). Parenting styles and substance use during childhood and adolescence. *Journal of Marriage and the Family, 50*, 473–482.

Cowan, P. A., Powell, D., & Cowan, C. P. (1998). Parenting interventions: A family systems perspective. In W. Damon (Series Ed.), I. E. Sigel & K. A. Renninger (Vol. Eds.), *Handbook of child psychology*, 5th ed., *Vol. 4, Child psychology in practice* (pp. 3–72). New York: Wiley.

Crick, N. R., & Dodge, K. A. (1994). A review and reformulation of social information-processing mechanisms in children's social adjustment. *Psychological Bulletin, 115*, 74–101.

Cross, W. (1990). Race and ethnicity: Effect on social networks. In M. Cochran, M. Larner, D. Riley, L. Gunnarson & C. R. Henderson (Eds.), *Extending families: The social networks of parents and their children* (pp. 67–85). Cambridge, England: Cambridge University Press.

Dance, K. A., & Neufeld, R. W. J. (1988). Aptitude-treatment interaction research in the clinical setting: A review of attempts to dispel the "patient uniformity" myth. *Psychological Bulletin, 104*, 192–213.

Daugherty, R. P., & Leukefeld, C. (1998). *Reducing the risks for substance abuse: A lifespan approach*. New York: Plenum.

Deater-Deckard, K., Dodge, K. A., Bates, J. E., & Pettit, G. S. (1996). Physical discipline among African-American and European-American mothers: Links to children's externalizing behaviors. *Developmental Psychology, 32*, 1065–1072.

DeGagni, G. A., Wietlisbach, S., Poisson, S., Stein, E., & Royeen, C. (1994). The impact of culture and socioeconomic status on family-professional collaboration: Challenges and solutions. *Topics in Early Childhood Education, 14*, 503–520.

Demo, D. H., Small, S. A., & Savin-Williams, R. C. (1987). Family relations and the self-esteem of adolescents and their parents. *Journal of Marriage and the Family, 49*, 705–715.

Dembo, M. H., & Gibson, S. (1985). Teachers' sense of efficacy: An important factor in school improvement. *The Elementary School Journal, 86*, 173–184.

Dinkmeyer, D., & McKay, G. (1976). *Systematic training for effective parenting (STEP)*. Circle Pines, MN: American Guidance Service.

Dishion, T. J. (1990). The family ecology of boys' peer relations in middle childhood. *Child Development, 61*, 109–117.

Dishion, T. J., McCord, J., & Poulin, F. (1999). When interventions harm: Peer groups and problem behavior. *American Psychologist, 54*, 755–764.

Dishion, T. J., Reid, J. G., & Patterson, G. R. (1988). Empirical guidelines for a family intervention for adolescent drug use. *Journal of Chemical Dependency Treatment, 1,* 189–224.

Dix, T. H., & Grusec, J. E. (1985). Parent attribution processes in the socialization of children. In I. E. Sigel (Ed.), *Parental belief systems: The psychological consequences for children* (pp. 201–233). Hillsdale, NJ: Erlbaum.

Dix, R., Reinhold, D. P., & Zambarano, R. J. (1990). Mothers' judgment in moments of anger. *Merrill-Palmer Quarterly, 36,* 465–486.

Dix, T. H., Ruble, D. N., & Zambarano, R. J. (1989). Mothers' implicit theories of discipline: Child effects, parent effects, and the attribution process. *Child Development, 60,* 1373–1391.

Djazair, R., Donovan, J. E., & Costa, F. M. (1991). *Beyond adolescence: Problem behavior and young adult development.* Cambridge, England: Cambridge University Press.

Dobkin, P. L., Tremblay, R. E., & Sacchitelle, C. (1997). Predicting boys' early-onset substance abuse from father's alcoholism, son's disruptiveness, and mother's parenting behavior. *Journal of Consulting and Clinical Psychology, 65,* 86–92.

Dodge, K. A. (1986). A social information processing model of social competence in children. In M. Perlmutter (Ed.), *The Minnesota Symposium on Child Psychology* (Vol. 18, pp. 77–125). Hillsdale, NJ: Erlbaum.

Drug Strategies. (1999). *Making the grade: A guide to school drug prevention programs.* Washington, DC: Author.

Dunn, J., & Plomin, R. (1991). Why are siblings so different? The significance of differences in sibling experience within the family. *Family Process, 30,* 271–283.

Dunst, C. J., & Trivette, C. M. (1990). Assessment of social support in early intervention programs. In S. J. Meisels & J. P. Shonkoff (Eds.), *Handbook of early childhood intervention* (pp. 326–349). Cambridge, England: Cambridge University Press.

Dweck, C. W., & Elliot, E. S. (1983). Achievement motivation. In P. H. Mussen (Series Ed.) & E. M. Hetherington (Vol. Ed.), *Handbook of child psychology* 4th ed., Vol. 4, *Socialization, personality, and social development* (pp. 643–692). New York: Wiley.

Eccles, J. S. (1993). School and family effects on the ontogeny of children's interests, self-perceptions, and activity choices. *Nebraska Symposium on Motivation, 40,* 145–208.

Efran, J. S., Greene, M. A., & Gordon, D. E. (1998). Lessons of the new genetics: Finding the right fit for our clients. *Family Therapy Networker,* 3–8, 11–17.

Eisen, M., Zellman, G. L., & McAllister, A. L. (1985). A Health Belief Model approach to adolescent fertility control: Some pilot program findings. *Health Education Quarterly, 12,* 185–210.

Eisenberg, N., & Fabes, R. A. (1998). Prosocial development. In W. Damon (Series Ed.) & N. Eisenberg (Vol. Ed.), *Handbook of child psychology,* 5th ed., Vol. 3, *Social, emotional, and personality development* (pp. 701–778). New York: Wiley.

Eisenberg, N., & Murphy, B. (1995). Parenting and children's moral development. In M. H. Bornstein (Ed.), *Handbook of parenting. Vol. 4, Applied and practical parenting* (pp. 227–257). Mahwah, NJ: Erlbaum.

Ellickson, P. L., Bell, R. M., & McGuigan, K. (1993). Preventing adolescent drug use: Long-term results of a junior high program. *American Journal of Public Health, 83,* 856–861.

Faber, A., & Mazlish, E. (1980). *How to talk so kids will listen & listen so kids will talk.* New York: Avon.

Feiring, C., & Taska, L. S. (1996). Family self-concept: Ideas on its meaning. In B. Bracken (Ed.), *Handbook of self-concept* (pp. 317–373). New York: Wiley.

Finkelstein, N. W., & Ramey, C. T. (1977). Learning to control the environment in infancy. *Child Development, 48,* 806–819.

Fritz, J., & MacPhee, D. (1991, April). *Enhancing at-risk parents' sense of competence.* Poster presented at the *Biennial Meeting of the Society for Research in Child Development,* Seattle.

Fritz, J., MacPhee, D., & Miller-Heyl, J. (1999, April). *Parent social cognitions and children's interpersonal problem solving*. Poster presented at the *Biennial Meeting of the Society for Research in Child Development*, Albuquerque, NM.

Fritz, J. J., Miller-Heyl, J., Kreutzer, J. C., & MacPhee, D. (1995). Fostering personal teaching efficacy through staff development and classroom activities. *Journal of Educational Research, 88*, 200–208.

Fuligni, A. J., & Eccles, J. S. (1993). Perceived parent–child relationships and early adolescents' orientation toward peers. *Developmental Psychology, 29*, 622–632.

Gallagher, J. J. (1990). The family as a focus for intervention. In S. J. Meisels & J. P. Shonkoff (Eds.), *Handbook of early childhood intervention* (pp. 540–559). Cambridge, England: Cambridge University Press.

Garbarino, J. (1992). *Children and families in the social environment*. Hawthorne, NY: Aldine de Gruyter.

Garbarino, J., & Sherman, D. (1980). High-risk neighborhoods and high-risk families: The human ecology of child maltreatment. *Child Development, 51*, 188–198.

Garmezy, N. (1989). The role of competence in the study of children and adolescents under stress. In E. Schneider, G. Attili, J. Nadel, & E. Weissberg (Eds.), *Social competence in developmental perspective* (pp. 25–39). Dordrecht, Netherlands: Kluwer.

Gelfand, D. M., & Teti, D. M. (1990). The effects of maternal depression on children. *Clinical Psychology Review, 10*, 329–353.

Gerard, A. B. (1994). *The Parent-Child Relationship Inventory: Manual*. Los Angeles: Western Psychological Services.

Gibson, S., & Dembo, M. H. (1984). Teacher efficacy: A construct validation. *Journal of Educational Psychology, 76*, 569–582.

Gilmartin, B. G. (1979). The case against spanking. *Human Behavior, 8*, 18–23.

Golding, J. M., & Baezconde-Garbanati, L. A. (1990). Ethnicity, culture, and social resources. *American Journal of Community Psychology, 18*, 465–486.

Goodman, S. H., & Gotlib, I. H. (1999). Risk for psychopathology in the children of depressed mothers: A developmental model for understanding mechanisms of transmission. *Psychological Review, 106*, 458–490.

Gottfried, A. W., Guerin, D., Spencer, J. E., & Meyer, C. (1984). Validity of the Minnesota Child Development Inventory in screening young children's developmental status. *Journal of Pediatric Psychology, 9*, 219–230.

Gottman, J. M., Coan, J., Carrere, S., & Swanson, C. (1998). Predicting marital happiness and stability from newlywed interactions. *Journal of Marriage and the Family, 60*, 5–22.

Greenwood, G. E., Olejnik, S. F., & Parkay, F. W. (1990). Relationships between four teacher efficacy belief patterns and selected teacher characteristics. *Journal of Research and Development in Education, 23*, 102–106.

Grover, P. L. (Ed.) (1998). *Preventing substance abuse among children and families: Family-centered approaches*. Rockville, MD: Substance Abuse and Mental Health Services Administration, Department of Health and Human Services (DHHS Publication No. 3223-FY98).

Guerin, D., & Gottfried, A. (1987). Minnesota Child Development Inventory: Predictors of intelligence, achievement, and adaptability. *Journal of Pediatric Psychology, 12*, 595–610.

Hahn, E. J., & Rado, M. (1996). African American Head Start parent involvement in drug prevention. *American Journal of Health Behavior, 20*, 41–51.

Hansen, W. (1997). Prevention programs: Factors that individually focused programs must address. In *Secretary's youth substance abuse prevention initiative: Resource papers* (pp. 53–66). Rockville, MD: Center for Substance Abuse Prevention, Substance Abuse and Mental Health Services Administration, Department of Health and Human Services.

Harris, J. R. (1998). *The nurture assumption: Why children turn out the way they do*. New York: Free Press.

Harrison, A. O., Wilson, M. N., Pine, C. J., Chan, S. Q., & Burie, R. (1990). Family ecologies of ethnic minority children. *Child Development, 61,* 347–362.

Harter, S. (1983). Developmental perspectives on the self-system. In P. H. Mussen (Series Ed.) & E. M. Hetherington (Vol. Ed.), *Handbook of child psychology,* 4th ed., *Vol. 4, Socialization, personality, and social development* (pp. 275–386). New York: Wiley.

Harter, S. (1992). Visions of self: Beyond the me in the mirror. In J. E. Jacobs (Ed.), *Developmental perspectives on motivation* (pp. 99–144). Lincoln, NE: University of Nebraska.

Harter, S. (1999). *The construction of the self: A developmental perspective.* New York: Guilford.

Hartup, W. W. (1989). Social relationships and their developmental significance. *American Psychologist, 44,* 120–126.

Haskett, M. E. (1990). Social problem-solving skills of young physically abused children. *Child Psychiatry and Human Development, 21,* 109–118.

Hawkins, J. D., Catalano, R. F., Jr., & Associates. (1992). *Communities that care: Action for drug abuse prevention.* San Francisco: Jossey-Bass.

Hawkins, J. D., Catalano, R., & Miller, J. (1992). Risk and protective factors for alcohol and other drug problems in adolescence and early adulthood: Implications for substance abuse prevention. *Psychological Bulletin, 112,* 64–105.

Henggeler, S. W., Melton, G. B., Brondino, M. J., Scherer, D. G., & Hanley, J. H. (1997). Multisystemic therapy with violent and chronic juvenile offenders and their families: The role of treatment fidelity in successful dissemination. *Journal of Consulting and Clinical Psychology, 65,* 821–833.

Hinde, R. A., & Tamplin, A. (1983). Relations between mother-child interaction and behavior in preschool. *British Journal of Developmental Psychology, 1,* 231–257.

Hinde, R., Tamplin, A., & Barrett, J. (1993). A comparative study of relationship structure. *British Journal of Social Psychology, 32,* 191–207.

Hoffman, M. L. (1984). Empathy, its limitations, and its role in a comprehensive moral theory. In W. M. Kurtines & J. L. Gewirtz (Eds.), *Morality, moral behavior, and moral development.* New York: Wiley.

Holmes, S. J., & Robins, L. N. (1988). The role of parental disciplinary practices in the development of depression and alcoholism. *Psychiatry, 51,* 24–35.

Hops, H., Tildesley, E., Lichtenstein, E., Ary, D., & Sherman, L. (1990). Parent-adolescent problem-solving interactions and drug use. *American Journal of Drug and Alcohol Abuse, 16,* 239–258.

Howard, M. O., Kivlahan, D., & Walker, R. D. (1997). Cloninger's tridimensional theory of personality and psychopathology: Applications to substance use disorders. *Journal of Studies on Alcohol, 58,* 48–66.

Ireton, H., & Thwing, E. (1974). *Manual for the Minnesota Child Development Inventory.* Minneapolis: Behavioral Science Systems.

Jackson, S., Bijstra, J., Oostra, L., & Bosma, H. (1998). Adolescents' perceptions of communication with parents relative to specific aspects of relationships with parents and personality development. *Journal of Adolescence, 21,* 305–322.

Jessor, R., Donovan, J. E., & Costa, F. M. (1991). *Beyond adolescence: Problem behavior and young adult development.* Cambridge, England: Cambridge University Press.

Johnson, D., & Walker, T. (1991). *Final report of an evaluation of the Avance parent education and family support program.* Report submitted to the Carnegie Corporation.

Jones, D. C., & Houts, R. (1992). Parental drinking, parent-child communication, and social skills in young adults. *Journal of Studies on Alcohol, 53,* 48–56.

Judd, V., & Forgues, C. (1989). Canada's homeless: Breaking down the barriers to health care. *The Canadian Nurse, 85*(10), 18–19.

Kafka, R. R., & London, P. (1991). Communication in relationships and adolescent substance use: The influence of parents and friends. *Adolescence, 26,* 587–598.

Kauffman, S., & Poulin, J. (1994). Citizen participation in prevention activities: A path model. *Journal of Consulting and Clinical Psychology, 65,* 453–463.

Kaufert, J. M. (1986). Health beliefs as predictors of success of alternative modalities of smoking cessation: Results of a controlled trial. *Journal of Behavioral Medicine, 9,* 475–489.

Kazdin, A. E., Holland, L., & Crowley, M. (1997). Family experience of barriers to treatment and premature termination from child therapy. *Journal of Consulting and Clinical Psychology, 65,* 453–463.

Keane, S. P., Brown, K. P., & Crenshaw, T. M. (1990). Children's intention-cue detection as a function of maternal social behavior: Pathways to social rejection. *Developmental Psychology, 26,* 1004–1009.

Kelley, M. A., Perlof, J. D., Morris, N. M., & Liu, W. (1992). The role of perceived barriers in the use of a comprehensive prenatal care program. *Journal of Health and Social Policy, 3,* 81–89.

Kieren, D. K., & Doherty-Poirier, M. (1993). Teaching about family communication and problem solving: Issues and future directions. In M. E. Arcus, J. D. Schvaneveldt, & J. J. Moss (Eds.), *Handbook of family life education. Vol. 2. The practice of family life education* (pp. 155–179). Newbury Park, CA: Sage.

King, J. A., Morris, L. L., & Fitz-Gibbon, C. T. (1987). *How to assess program implementation.* Newbury Park, CA: Sage.

Klein, K., Forehand, R., Armistead, L., & Long, P. (1997). Delinquency during the transition to early adulthood: Family and parenting predictors from early adolescence. *Adolescence, 32,* 61–80.

Knight, G. P., Virdin, L. M., & Roosa, M. (1994). Socialization and family correlates of mental health outcomes among Hispanic and Anglo-American children: Consideration of cross-ethnic scalar equivalence. *Child Development, 65,* 212–224.

Kohlberg, L. (1976). Moral stages and moralization: The cognitive-developmental approach. In T. Lickona (Ed.), *Moral development and behavior: Theory, research, and social issues* (pp. 31–53). New York: Holt, Rinehart & Winston.

Kohlberg, L. (1984). *Essays on moral development: The psychology of moral development.* New York: Harper & Row.

Kretzmann, J. P., & McKnight, J. L. (1993). *Building communities from the inside out: A path toward finding and mobilizing a community's assets.* Chicago: ACTA Publications.

Kumpfer, K. L., & Alvarado, R. (1995). Strengthening families to prevent drug use in multi-ethnic youth. In G. Botvin, S. Schinke, & M. Orlando (Eds.), *Drug abuse prevention in multi-ethnic youth* (pp. 255–294). Thousand Oaks, CA: Sage.

Kupersmidt, J. B., & Coie, J. D. (1990). Preadolescent peer status, aggression, and school adjustment as predictors of externalizing problems in adolescence. *Child Development, 61,* 1350–1362.

Kurdek, L. A. (1982). Long-term predictive validity of children's social-cognitive assessments. *Merrill-Palmer Quarterly, 28,* 511–521.

Ladd, G. W., & Golter, B. S. (1988). Parents' management of preschoolers' peer relations: Is it related to children's social competence? *Developmental Psychology, 24,* 109–117.

Larrance, D. T., & Twentyman, C. T. (1983). Maternal attributions in child abuse. *Journal of Abnormal Psychology, 92,* 449–457.

Lazar, I., & Darlington, R. (1982). Lasting effects of early education: A report from the Consortium for Longitudinal Studies. *Monographs of the Society for Research in Child Development, 47* (Serial No. 195).

Lepper, M. R. (1983). Social-control processes and the internalization of social values: An attributional perspective. In E. T. Higgins, D. N. Ruble, & W. W. Hartup (Eds.), *Social cognition and social development* (pp. 294–330). Cambridge, England: Cambridge University Press.

Levenson, H. (1974). Activism and powerful others: distinctions within the concept of internal-external control. *Journal of Personality Assessment, 38,* 377–383.

Levenson, H. (1981). Differentiating among internality, powerful others, and chance. In H. M. Lefcourt

(Ed.), *Research with the locus of control construct: Vol. 1, Assessment methods* (pp. 15–63). Orlando: Academic Press.

LeVine, R. A. (1988). Human parental care: Universal goals, cultural strategies, individual behavior. *New Directions for Child Development, 40,* 3–12.

Levitt, M. J., Guacci-Franco, N., & Levitt, J. L. (1993). Convoys of social support in childhood and early adolescence: Structure and function. *Developmental Psychology 29,* 811–818.

Levitt, M. J., Weber, R. A., & Clark, M. C. (1986). Social network relationships as sources of maternal support and well-being. *Developmental Psychology, 22,* 310–316.

Loeber, R., & Dishion, T. (1983). Early predictors of male delinquency: A review. *Psychological Bulletin, 94,* 68–99.

Loeber, R., Green, S. M., Keenan, K., & Lahey, B. B. (1995). Which boys will fare worse? Early predictors of the onset of conduct disorder in a six-year longitudinal study. *Journal of the American Academy of Child and Adolescent Psychiatry, 34,* 499–509.

LoSciuto, L., Rajala, A. K., Townsend, T. N., & Taylor, A. S. (1996). An outcome evaluation of Across Ages: An intergenerational mentoring approach to drug prevention. *Journal of Adolescent Research, 11,* 116–129.

MacPhee, D. (1986, April). *The measurement of difficult child behavior.* Poster presented at the *Biennial International Conference on Infant Studies,* Los Angeles.

MacPhee, D. (1999). Prevention. In C. A. Smith (Ed.), *The encyclopedia of parenting theory and research* (pp. 336–338). Westport, CT: Greenwood.

MacPhee, D., Benson, J. B., & Bullock, D. (1986, April). *Influences on maternal self-perceptions.* Poster presented at the *Biennial International Conference on Infant Studies,* Los Angeles.

MacPhee, D., Fritz, J., & Miller-Heyl, J. (1996). Ethnic variations in personal social networks and parenting. *Child Development, 67,* 3278–3295.

MacPhee, D., & Rattenborg, K. (1991, April). *Cognitive mediators of child abuse.* Poster presented at the *Biennial Meeting of the Society for Research in Child Development,* Seattle.

MacQueen, A. R. (1999). Spiritual dimensions of alcohol and other drug problems. *Addiction, 9,* 436.

Mantzicopoulos, P. Y. (1997). The relationship of family variables to Head Start children's pre-academic competence. *Early Education and Development, 8,* 357–375.

Markus, H., Cross, S., & Wurf, E. (1990). The role of the self-system in competence. In R. Sternberg & J. Kolligian (Eds.), *Competence considered* (pp. 205–226). New Haven, CT: Yale University.

Marshall, W. L., & Serin, R. (1997). Personality disorders. In S. M. Turner & M. Hersen (Eds.), *Adult psychopathology and diagnosis* (3rd ed., pp. 508–543). New York: Wiley.

Martinez, E. (1993). Parenting young children in Mexican-American/Chicano families. In H. P. McAdoo (Ed.), *Family ethnicity* (pp. 184–195). Newbury Park, CA: Sage.

McBride, D. C., Mutch, P. B., & Chitwood, D. D. (1996). Religious belief and the initiation and prevention of drug use among youth. In C. B. McCoy, L. R. Metsch, & J. A. Inciardi (Eds.), *Intervening with drug-involved youth* (pp. 110–130). Thousand Oaks, CA: Sage.

McGrew, J. H., Bond, G. R., Dietzen, L., & Salyers, M. (1994). Measuring the fidelity of implementation of a mental health program model. *Journal of Consulting and Clinical Psychology, 62,* 670–678.

McLoyd, V. C. (1990). Impact of economic hardship on Black families and children: Psychological distress, parenting, and socioemotional development. *Child Development, 61,* 311–346.

Miller[-Heyl], J. L. (1981). *Impact of DARE to be You program on 8–12-year-old youth as they become 10–14-years old.* Final Report to Centers for Disease Control, Atlanta, GA.

Miller-Heyl, J., MacPhee, D., & Fritz, J. J., (1998). DARE to be You: A family-support, early prevention program. *Journal of Primary Prevention, 18,* 257–285.

Minuchin, P. P. (1985). Families and individual development: Provocations from the field of family therapy. *Child Development, 56,* 289–302.

Moffitt, T. E. (1993). Adolescence-limited and life-course-persistent antisocial behavior: A developmental taxonomy. *Psychological Review, 100*, 674–701.

Moos, R. H., & Trickett, E. J. (1987). *Classroom Environment Scale* (2nd ed.). Palo Alto, CA: Consulting Psychologists Press.

Morison, P., & Masten, A. S. (1991). Peer reputation in middle childhood as a predictor of adaptation in adolescence: A seven-year follow-up. *Child Development, 62*, 991–1007.

National Research Council. (1993). *Losing generations: Adolescents in high-risk settings*. Washington, DC: National Academy Press.

Nelson, S. A. (1980). Factors influencing young children's use of motives and outcomes as moral criteria. *Child Development, 51*, 823–829.

Newcomb, A. F., & Bagwell, C. L. (1996). The developmental significance of children's friendship relations. In W. M. Bukowski, A. F. Newcomb, & W. W. Hartup (Eds.), *The company they keep: Friendship in childhood and adolescence* (pp. 289–321). Cambridge, England: Cambridge University Press.

NICHD Early Child Care Research Network. (1999). Child outcomes when child care center classes meet recommended standards for quality. *American Journal of Public Health, 89*, 1072–1077.

Nichols, M. P., & Schwartz, R. C. (1995). *Family therapy: Concepts and methods* (3rd ed.). New York: Allyn and Bacon.

Nix, R. L., Pinderhughes, E. E., Dodge, K. A., Bates, J. E., Pettit, G. S., & McFadyen-Ketchum, S. A. (1999). The relation between mothers' hostile attribution tendencies and children's externalizing behavior problems: The mediating role of mothers' harsh discipline practices. *Child Development, 70*, 896–909.

Northam, S. (1996). Access to health promotion, protection, and disease prevention among impoverished individuals. *Public Health Nursing, 13*, 353–364.

Nurmi, J. E. (1993). Adolescent development in an age-graded context: The role of personal beliefs, goals, and strategies in the tackling of developmental tasks and standards. *International Journal of Behavioral Development, 16*, 169–189.

Odum, H. T. (1971). *Environment, power, and society*. New York: Wiley.

Oetting, G., & Beauvais, F. (1987). Peer cluster theory, socialization characteristics, and adolescent drug use: A path analysis. *Journal of Consulting Psychology, 34*, 205–213.

Olds, D. (1997). The Prenatal/Early Infancy Project: Fifteen years later. In G. W. Albee & T. P. Gullotta (Eds.), *Primary prevention works* (pp. 41–67). Thousand Oaks, CA: Sage.

Olds, D. L., Henderson, C. R., Tatelbaum, R., & Chamberlin, R. (1986). Preventing child abuse and neglect: A randomized trial of nurse home visitation. *Pediatrics, 78*, 65–78.

Owens, C. J. (1994). *The impact of access to transportation on appointment keeping behavior in a community mental health agency*. Unpublished doctoral dissertation, California School of Professional Psychology, Los Angeles, CA.

Ozer, E. M., & Bandura, A. (1990). Mechanisms governing empowerment effects: A self-efficacy analysis. *Journal of Personality and Social Psychology, 58*, 472–486.

Parke, R. D., & Ladd, G. W. (1992). *Family-peer relationships: Modes of linkage*. Hillsdale, NJ: Erlbaum.

Patterson, G. R., DeBaryshe, B. D., & Ramsey, E. (1989). A developmental perspective on antisocial behavior. *American Psychologist, 44*, 329–335.

Patterson, G., Reid, J., & Dishion, T. (1992). *Antisocial boys*. Eugene, OR: Castalia.

Peisner-Feinberg, E., & Burchinal, M. R. (1997). Relations between children's child-care experiences and concurrent development: The Cost, Quality, and Outcomes Study. *Merrill-Palmer Quarterly, 43*, 451–477.

Pettit, J. (1990). *Utes: The mountain people (Rev. ed.)*. Boulder, CO. Johnson.

Piaget, J. (1965). *The moral judgment of the child*. New York: Free Press.

Pianta, R., Egeland, B., & Sroufe, L. A. (1990). Maternal stress and children's development: Prediction of school outcomes and identification of protective factors. In J. E. Rolf, A. S. Masten, D. Cicchetti, K. Nuechterlein, & S. Weintraub (Eds.), *Risk and protective factors in the development of psychopathology* (pp. 215–235). Cambridge, England: Cambridge University Press.

Plomin, R., DeFries, J., & Loehlin, J. (1977). Genotype-environment interaction and correlation in the analysis of human development. *Psychological Bulletin, 84,* 309–322.

Plomin, R., & McClearn, G. E. (Eds.). (1993). *Nature, nurture, and psychology.* Washington, DC: American Psychological Association.

Price, R. H., Cowen, E. L., Lorion, R. P., & Ramos-McKay, J. (1989). The search for effective prevention programs: What we learned along the way. *American Journal of Orthopsychiatry, 59,* 49–58.

Quintana, F. L. (1991). *Pobladores: Hispanic-Americans of the Ute frontier.* Notre Dame, IN: University of Notre Dame Press.

Rees, C. D., & Wilborn, B. L. (1983). Correlates of drug use in adolescents: A comparison of families of drug abusers with families of nondrug abusers. *Journal of Youth and Adolescence, 12,* 55–63.

Reis, J. (1996). A descriptive study of African-American mother-child communication about drugs and health. *Journal of Comparative Family Studies, 27,* 485–498.

Resnick, G. (1985). Enhancing parental competencies for high risk mothers: An evaluation of prevention effects. *Child Abuse & Neglect, 9,* 479–489.

Reynolds, R., Stewart, K., & Fisher, D. (1997). A framework for prevention: Science and practice in action. In *Secretary's youth substance abuse prevention initiative: Resource papers* (pp. 1–14). Rockville, MD: Center for Substance Abuse Prevention, Substance Abuse and Mental Health Services Administration, U.S. Department of Health and Human Services.

Rhodes, J., & Jason, L. (1990). A social stress model of substance abuse. *Journal of Consulting and Clinical Psychology, 58,* 395–401.

Rist, R. (1970). Student social class and teacher expectations: Fulfilling prophecy in ghetto education. *Harvard Educational Review, 40,* 411–451.

Roberts, R. N., Wasik, B. H., Casto, G., & Ramey, C. T. (1991). Family support in the home: Programs, policy, and social change. *American Psychologist, 46,* 131–137.

Robertson, D. L., & Reynolds, A. J. (1999, April). *Family typologies and child educational outcomes: Are they related?* Paper presented at the *Biennial Meeting of the Society for Research in Child Development,* Albuquerque, NM.

Roopnarine, J. L. (1987). Social interaction in the peer group: Relationship to perceptions of parenting and to children's interpersonal awareness and problem-solving ability. *Journal of Applied Developmental Psychology, 8,* 351–362.

Rosenberg, M. S., & Reppucci, N. D. (1985). Primary prevention of child abuse. *Journal of Consulting and Clinical Psychology, 53,* 576–585.

Rossi, P. H., & Freeman, H. E. (1989). *Evaluation: A systematic approach* (4th ed.). Newbury Park, CA: Sage.

Rotheram-Borus, M. J., & Koopman, C. (1990). AIDS and adolescence. In R. Lerner, A. Peterson, & J. Brooks-Gunn (Eds.), *Encyclopedia of adolescence* (pp. 29–36). New York: Garland.

Rotter, J. (1966). Generalized expectancies for internal versus external control of reinforcement. *Psychological Monographs: General and Applied, 80* (Whole No. 609), 1–28.

Rowe, D. C., & Rodgers, J. L. (1989). Behavioral genetics, adolescent deviance, and "d": Contributions and issues. In G. R. Adams, R. Montemayor, & T. P. Gullotta (Eds.), *Biology of adolescent behavior and development* (pp. 71–97). Newbury Park, CA: Sage.

Rubin, K. H., Mills, R., & Rose-Krasnor, L. (1989). Maternal beliefs and children's competence. In B. H. Schneider, G. Attili, J. Nadel, & R. P. Weissberg (Eds.), *Social competence in developmental perspective* (pp. 313–331). Dordrecht, Netherlands: Kluwer.

Rutter, M. (1979). Protective factors in children's responses to stress and disadvantage. In M. W. Kent

& J. E. Rolf (Eds.), *Primary prevention of psychopathology: Vol. 3, Social competence in children* (pp. 49–74). Hanover, NH: University Press of New England.

Rutter, M. (1983a). School effects on pupil progress: Research findings and policy implications. *Child Development, 54,* 1–29.

Rutter, M. (1983b). Stress, coping, and development: Some issues and some questions. In N. Garmezy & M. Rutter (Eds.), *Stress, coping and development* (pp. 1–42). Baltimore, MD: Johns Hopkins University Press.

Rutter, M. (1990). Psychological risk and protective mechanisms. In J. E. Rolf, A. S. Masten, D. Cicchetti, K. Nuechterlein, & S. Weintraub (Eds.), *Risk and protective factors in the development of psychopathology* (pp. 181–214). Cambridge, England: Cambridge University Press.

Sameroff, A. J., & Seifer, R. (1983). Familial risk and child competence. *Child Development, 54,* 1254–1268.

Scales, P. (1990). Developing capable young people: An alternative strategy for prevention programs. *Journal of Early Adolescence, 10,* 420–438.

Schorr, L. (1989). *Within our reach.* New York: Avon.

Scott-Jones, D. (1995). Parent-child interactions and school achievement. In B. A. Ryan, G. R. Adams, T. P. Gullotta, R. P. Weisberg, & R. L. Hampton (Eds.). *The family-school connection: Theory, research and practice* (pp. 75–107). Thousand Oaks, CA: Sage.

Seligman, M. E. P. (1975). *Helplessness.* San Francisco: Freeman.

Seligman, M. E. P. (1995). *The optimistic child.* Boston: Houghton Mifflin.

Selman, R. L. (1980). *The growth of interpersonal understanding.* New York: Academic.

Seybold, J., Fritz, J., & MacPhee, D. (1991). Relation of social support to self-perceptions of mothers with delayed children. *Journal of Community Psychology, 19,* 29–36.

Shaffer, D. R. (1988). *Social and personality development,* 2nd ed. Belmont, CA: Brooks/Cole.

Shaffer, D. R. (2000). *Social and personality development,* 4th ed. Belmont, CA: Wadsworth.

Shern, D. L., Trochim, W. M. K., & LaComb, C. A. (1995). The use of concept mapping for assessing fidelity of model transfer: An example from psychiatric rehabilitation. *Evaluation and Program Planning, 12,* 1–16.

Shoham-Salomon, V., & Hannah, M. T. (1991). Client-treatment interaction in the study of differential change processes. *Journal of Consulting and Clinical Psychology, 59,* 217–225.

Shure, M. B., & Spivak, G. (1982). Interpersonal problem solving in young children: A cognitive approach to prevention. *American Journal of Community Psychology, 10,* 341–356.

Shure, M. B. (1997). Interpersonal cognitive problem solving: Primary prevention of early high-risk behaviors in preschool and primary years. In G. W. Albee & T. P. Gullotta (Eds.), *Primary prevention works: Vol. 6, Issues in children's families' lives.* Thousand Oaks, CA; Sage.

Siegal, M., & Peterson, C. C. (1998). Preschoolers' understanding of lies and innocent and negligent mistakes. *Developmental Psychology, 34,* 332–341.

Sirignano, S. W., & Lachman, M. E. (1985). Personality change during the transition to parenthood: The role of perceived infant temperament. *Developmental Psychology, 21,* 558–567.

Slaughter, D. T. (1988). Programs for racially and ethnically diverse American families: Some critical issues. In H. B. Weiss & F. H. Jacobs (Eds.), *Evaluating family programs* (pp. 461–476). New York: Aldine de Gruyter.

Slonim-Nevo, V., Ozawa, M. N., & Auslander, W. F. (1991). Knowledge, attitudes, and behavior related to AIDS among youth in residential centers: Results from an exploratory study. *Journal of Adolescence, 14,* 17–33.

Smetana, J. G., Schlagman, N., & Adams, P. W. (1993). Preschool children's judgments about hypothetical and actual transgressions. *Child Development, 67,* 1153–1172.

Soderlund, J., Epstein, M. H., Quinn, K. P., Cumblad, C., & Petersen, S. (1995). Parental perspectives on comprehensive services for children and youth with emotional and behavioral disorders. *Behavioral Disorders, 20,* 157–170.

Spivak, G., & Shure, M. (1989). Interpersonal cognitive problem-solving (ICPS): A competence-building primary prevention program. *Prevention in Human Services, 6,* 151–178.

Spoth, R., Redmond, C., Haggerty, K., & Ward, T. (1995). A controlled parenting skills outcome study examining individual differences and attendance effects. *Journal of Marriage and the Family, 57,* 449–464.

Stafford, L., & Bayer, C. L. (1993). *Interaction between parents and children.* Newbury Park, CA: Sage.

Steele, C. M. (1997). A threat in the air: How stereotypes shape intellectual identity and performance. *American Psychologist, 52,* 613–629.

Steinberg, L., Darling, N. E., & Fletcher, A. C. (1995). Authoritative parenting and adolescent adjustment: An ecological journey. In P. Moen, G. H. Elder, Jr., & K. Luscher (Eds.), *Examining lives in context: Perspectives on the ecology of human development* (pp. 423–466). Washington, DC: American Psychological Association.

Strassberg, Z. (1995). Social information processing in compliance situations by mothers of behavior-problem boys. *Child Development, 66,* 376–389.

Sturner, R. A., Funk, S. G., Thomas, P. D., & Green, J. A. (1982). An adaptation of the Minnesota Child Development Inventory for preschool developmental screening. *Journal of Pediatric Psychology, 7,* 295–306.

Super, C. M., & Harkness, S. (1986). The developmental niche. A conceptualization of the interface of child and culture. *International Journal of Behavioral Development, 9,* 546–569.

Taylor, A., & Dryfoos, J. (1999). Creating a safe passage: Elder mentors and vulnerable youth. *Generations, 22*(4), 43–48.

Teti, D. M., & Gelfand, D. M. (1991). Behavioral competence among mothers of infants in the first year: The mediational role of maternal self-efficacy. *Child Development, 62,* 918–929.

Teti, D. M., O'Connell, M. A., & Reiner, C. D. (1996). Parenting sensitivity, parental depression and child health: The mediational role of parental self-efficacy. *Early Development & Parenting, 5,* 237–250.

Tietjen, A. (1994). Supportive interactions in cultural context. In F. Nestmann & K. Hurrelmann (Eds.), *Social networks and social support in childhood and adolescence* (pp. 395–408). New York: Aldine de Gruyter.

Triandis, H. C. (1995). *Individualism and collectivism.* Boulder, CO: Westview.

Trochim, W. M. K. (1989). An introduction to concept mapping for planning and evaluation. *Evaluation and Program Planning, 12,* 1–16.

Turner, H. A., & Finkelhor, D. (1996). Corporal punishment as a stressor among youth. *Journal of Marriage and the Family, 58,* 155–166.

Unger, D. G., & Powell, D. H. (1980). Supporting families under stress: The role of social networks. *Family Relations, 29,* 566–574.

von Bertalanffy, L. (1981). *A systems view of man.* Boulder, CO: Westview Press.

Voydanoff, P., & Donnelly, B. W. (1998). Parents' risk and protective factors as predictors of parental well-being and behavior. *Journal of Marriage and the Family, 60,* 344–355.

Wasik, B. H., Ramey, C. T., Bryant, D. M., & Sparling, J. J. (1990). A longitudinal study of two early intervention strategies: Project CARE. *Child Development, 61,* 1682–1696.

Watson, C. G., Hancock, M., Gearhart, L. P., Malhovrh, P., Mendez, C., & Raden, M. (1997). A comparison of symptoms associated with early and late onset alcohol dependence. *Journal of Nervous and Mental Disease, 185,* 507–509.

Watzlawick, P., Beavin, J. H., & Jackson, D. D. (1967). *Pragmatics of human communication: A study of interaction patterns, pathologies, and paradoxes.* New York: Norton.

Webster-Stratton, C. (1992). *The incredible years: A trouble-shooting guide for parents of children aged 3–8.* Toronto: Umbrella Press.

Webster-Stratton, C., & Herbert, M. (1993). What really happens in parent training? *Behavior Modification, 17,* 407–456.

Weiner, B. (1986). *An attributional theory of motivation and emotion.* New York: Springer–Verlag.

Weinstein, R. S., Marshall, H. H., Sharp, L., & Botkin, M. (1987). Pygmalion and the students: Age and classroom differences in awareness of teacher expectations. *Child Development, 58,* 1079–1093.

Werner, E. E. (1990). Protective factors and individual resilience. In S. J. Meisels & J. P. Shonkoff (Eds.), *Handbook of early childhood intervention* (pp. 97–116). Cambridge, England: Cambridge University Press.

White, K. J., & Kistner, J. (1992). The influence of teacher feedback on young children's peer preferences and perceptions. *Developmental Psychology, 28,* 933–940.

Whitehurst, G. J., Arnold, D. C., Epstein, J. M., & Angell, A. L. (1994). A picture book reading intervention in day care and home for children from low-income families. *Developmental Psychology, 30,* 679–689.

Winter, M. M., & McDonald, D. C. (1997). Parents as teachers: Investing in good beginnings for children. In G. W. Albee & T. P. Gullotta (Eds.), *Primary prevention works* (pp. 119–145). Newbury Park, CA: Sage.

Wood, J. R. (1998). *Factors influencing the effectiveness of a family intervention for adolescent versus adult mothers.* Unpublished master's thesis, Colorado State University.

Woodward, A. M., Dwinell, A. D., & Arons, B. S. (1992). Barriers to mental health care for Hispanic-Americans: A literature review and discussion. *Journal of Mental Health Administration, 19,* 224–236.

Woolfolk, A., & Hoy, W. (1990). Prospective teachers' sense of efficacy and beliefs about control. *Journal of Educational Psychology, 82,* 81–91.

Yoshikawa, H. (1994). Prevention as cumulative protection: Effects of early family support and education on chronic delinquency and its risks. *Psychological Bulletin, 115,* 28–54.

Zahn-Waxler, C., Radke-Yarrow, M., & King, R. A. (1979). Child rearing and children's prosocial initiations toward victims of distress. *Child Development, 50,* 319–330.

Zimmerman, B. J. (1995). Self-efficacy and educational development. In A. Bandura (Ed.), *Self-efficacy in changing societies* (pp. 202–231). Cambridge, England: Cambridge University Press.

Zucker, R. A., Fitzgerald, H. E., & Moses, H. D. (1995). Emergence of alcohol problems and the several alcoholisms: A developmental perspective on etiologic theory and life course trajectory. In D. Cicchetti & D. J. Cohen (Eds.), *Developmental psychopathology* (pp. 677–711). New York: Wiley.

Index